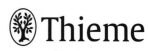

Venous Thromboembolism

A Practical Guide in Interventional Radiology

Jeffrey Weinstein, MD, FSIR
Assistant Professor of Radiology
Harvard Medical School, Beth Israel Deaconess Medical Center
Boston, Massachusetts, USA

Jeet Minocha, MD, FSIR
Chief of Vascular and Interventional Radiology and Associate Professor
Department of Radiology, University of California San Diego School of Medicine
La Jolla, California, USA

Joshua D. Dowell, MD, PhD, FSIR
Interventional Radiologist
Vascular and Interventional Physicians (VIP)
Northwest Radiology
Indianapolis, Indiana, USA

Series editor

Salomão Faintuch, MD, FSIR
Clinical Director of Interventional Radiology
Harvard Medical Faculty Physicians
Boston, Massachusetts, USA

91 Illustrations

Thieme
New York • Stuttgart • Delhi • Rio de Janeiro

Library of Congress Cataloging-in-Publication Data is available from the publisher.

Important note: Medicine is an ever-changing science undergoing continual development. Research and clinical experience are continually expanding our knowledge, in particular our knowledge of proper treatment and drug therapy. Insofar as this book mentions any dosage or application, readers may rest assured that the authors, editors, and publishers have made every effort to ensure that such references are in accordance with **the state of knowledge at the time of production of the book.**

Nevertheless, this does not involve, imply, or express any guarantee or responsibility on the part of the publishers in respect to any dosage instructions and forms of applications stated in the book. **Every user is requested to examine carefully** the manufacturers' leaflets accompanying each drug and to check, if necessary, in consultation with a physician or specialist, whether the dosage schedules mentioned therein or the contraindications stated by the manufacturers differ from the statements made in the present book. Such examination is particularly important with drugs that are either rarely used or have been newly released on the market. Every dosage schedule or every form of application used is entirely at the user's own risk and responsibility. The authors and publishers request every user to report to the publishers any discrepancies or inaccuracies noticed. If errors in this work are found after publication, errata will be posted at www.thieme.com on the product description page.

Some of the product names, patents, and registered designs referred to in this book are in fact registered trademarks or proprietary names even though specific reference to this fact is not always made in the text. Therefore, the appearance of a name without designation as proprietary is not to be construed as a representation by the publisher that it is in the public domain.

Thieme addresses people of all gender identities equally. We encourage our authors to use gender-neutral or gender-equal expressions wherever the context allows.

Thieme Publishers New York
333 Seventh Avenue, 18th Floor
New York, NY 10001, USA
www.thieme.com
+1 800 782 3488, customerservice@thieme.com

Cover design: © Thieme
Cover image source: © Matthieu/stock.adobe.com
Typesetting by TNQ Tech Private Limited, India

Printed in India by Replika Press Pvt. Ltd.   5 4 3 2 1

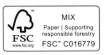

DOI: 10.1055/b-006-160168

ISBN: 978-1-62623-604-2

Also available as an e-book:
eISBN (PDF): 978-1-62623-605-9
eISBN (epub): 978-1-63853-482-2

Contents

10. Venous Thromboembolism: Management of Bleeding Complications

James Chen and Deepak Sudheendra

Foreword

I am honored to write this foreword for *Venous Thromboembolism: A Practical Guide in Interventional Radiology*. As the management of patients with venous thromboembolism (VTE) evolves, interventional radiology (IR) is at the forefront. While VTE, including deep vein thrombosis and pulmonary embolism, is common diagnosis, the approach to management varies based on several factors. The factors include everything from the severity of the thrombosis to its location and the patient's underlying risk factors for developing VTE.

Drs. Jeffrey Weinstein, Jeet Minocha, and Joshua D. Dowell have selected excellent leaders and experts in the field to contribute to this work. The book begins with the basics of pathogenesis, patient diagnosis, and medical therapies; all vital information for IRs to treat patients with VTE effectively. Chapters 4 to 9 guide the reader through patient selection and workup, basic and complex interventional techniques, and management of potential complications in a practical manner for a variety of pathologies and interventions (e.g., acute DVT, IVC filter management, chronic venous recanalization, pulmonary embolism, etc.). The authors also make note of current trials and publications with outcomes data throughout the text. The book is written with scientific integrity and in accessible language, making it a perfect resource for educating clinicians and resulting in improved clinical decision-making and procedural success.

Venous Thromboembolism: A Practical Guide in Interventional Radiology is a high-yield book that is a must-read for IRs who continue to be intricately involved with the management of patients with deep venous disease.

Minhaj S. Khaja, MD, MBA, FSIR
David M. Williams Research Professor
Professor of Radiology & Cardiac Surgery
Division of Vascular & Interventional Radiology
University of Michigan Health, Michigan, USA

Contributors

John Fritz Angle, M.D.
Professor of Radiology
Department Of Radiology
University of Virginia
Charlottesville, Virginia, USA

Kenneth A. Bauer, MD
Professor
Department of Medicine
Harvard Medical School
Boston, Massachusetts, USA

Olga R. Brook, MD, MBA
Section Chief of Abdominal Radiology
Department of Radiology
Beth Israel Deaconess Medical Center
Boston, Massachusetts, USA

Julie C. Bulman, MD
Interventional Radiologist
Department of Radiology
Harvard Medical School, Beth Israel Deaconess
    Medical Center
Boston, Massachusetts, USA

Brian J. Carney, MD
Assistant Professor
Department of Medicine
Harvard Medical School;
Medical Director of Apheresis Services
Department of Hematology and
    Hematologic Malignancies
Beth Israel Deaconess Medical Center
Boston, Massachusetts, USA

James Chen, MD
Vascular & Interventional Radiology
Charlotte Radiology
Charlotte, North Carolina, USA

Harika Dabbara, BS
Medical Student
Boston University Chobanian and
    Avedisian School of Medicine
Boston, Massachusetts, USA

Kush R. Desai, MD, FSIR
Associate Professor of Radiology,
    Surgery, and Medicine
Department oF Radiology
Northwestern University Feinberg
    School of Medicine
Chicago, Illinois, USA

Joshua D. Dowell, MD, PhD, FSIR
Interventional Radiologist
Northwest Radiology
Indianapolis, Indiana, USA

Salomão Faintuch, MD, FSIR
Clinical Director of Interventional Radiology
Harvard Medical Faculty Physicians
Boston, Massachusetts, USA

Karan S. Gulaya,MD, MPH
Attending Interventional Radiologist
Interventional Radiology
Radiology Associates of San Luis Obispo
San Luis Obispo, California, USA

David Heister, MD PhD
Interventional Radiologist
Department of Interventional Radiology
Baptist Health Medical Center
Little Rock, Arizona, USA

Mamdouh Khayat, MD
Vascular & Interventional Radiologist
Vascular & Interventional Radiology
Vive Vascular
Columbus, Ohio, USA

Alexander Y. Kim, MD, FSIR
Co-Founder and Medical Director
Department of Interventional Radiology
National Vascular Physicians
National Harbor, Maryland, USA

Thomas B. Kinney, MD, MSME
Emeritus Professor of Radiology
Department of Interventional Radiology
University of California-San Diego;
Interventional Radiologist
Department of Radiology
Naval Medical Center-San Diego
San Diego, California, USA

Robert J. Lewandowski, MD, FSIR
Professor of Radiology, Medicine, and Surgery;
Director of Interventional Oncology
Northwestern University Feinberg
    School of Medicine
Chicago, Illinois, USA

Mina S. Makary, MD
Interventional and Diagnostic Radiologist
Division of Vascular and Interventional Radiology
Department of Radiology
The Ohio State University Medical Center
Columbus, Ohio, USA

Shaun W. McLaughlin, MD, MS
Assistant Professor
Department of Interventional Radiology
Geisinger Health System
Wilkes-Barre, Pennsylvania, USA

Loren Mead, BA, MD
Staff Physician
Department of Emergency Medicine
UT Health Houston
Houston, Texas, USA

Jeet Minocha, MD, FSIR
Chief of Vascular and Interventional
    Radiology and Associate Professor
Department of Radiology
University of California San Diego
    School of Medicine
La Jolla, California, USA

Boris Nikolic, MD, MBA
Department of Radiology
Montefiore Nyack Hospital
New York, New York, USA

Scott Resnick, MD, FSIR
Professor of Radiology and Surgery
Northwestern University
Feinberg School of Medicine
Chicago, Illinois, USA

Dana Safavian, MD
Interventional Radiologist
Interventional Radiology
Brigham and Women's Hospital Harvard
    Medical School
Boston, Massachusetts, USA

Deepak Sudheendra, MD, MHCI, RPVI, FSIR
CEO and Medical Director
360 Vascular Institute
Dublin, Ohio, USA

Jeffrey Weinstein, MD, FSIR
Assistant Professor of Radiology
Harvard Medical School, Beth Israel Deaconess
    Medical Center
Boston, Massachusetts, USA

Nicholas Xiao, MD
Interventional Radiology Resident
Feinberg School of Medicine
Northwestern University
Chicago, Illinois, USA

Chapter 1

Introduction

1 Introduction

Harika Dabbara and Julie C. Bulman

Keywords: venous thromboembolism, incidence, mortality, PERT

Venous thromboembolism (VTE), constituted of deep vein thrombosis (DVT) and pulmonary embolism (PE), is a clinically morbid and highly prevalent chronic illness. Although precise numbers of individuals affected by VTE is not tracked, epidemiological analyses estimate an incidence between 1 and 2 individuals per 1,000 every year or 300,000 to 600,000 individuals are affected annually in the United States (▶ Fig. 1.1).[1,2,3] However, this incidence rate varies based on age, race, and gender.[1,4] In individuals older than 80 years, the incidence rises to 1 in 100 individuals (▶ Fig. 1.2). Men have a slightly higher incidence than women, aside from women in reproductive years, and the overall incidence is higher in black and white individuals than in other races.[1,4] Although most events are unprovoked, cancer and perioperative patients are at an increased risk. VTE can also often be fatal, with an estimated 25% of PE cases presenting with sudden death and all VTE carrying a 10 to 30% mortality rate within 30 days.[1] Given this high incidence, VTE imposes a considerable economic burden, costing $7,594 to $16,644 per patient and an annual cost of $2 to $10 billion.[1,5] Furthermore, it is the leading preventable cause of in-hospital mortality in the United States.[6]

Diagnosing VTE based on clinical symptoms is generally unreliable due to nonspecific signs. Clinical symptoms of DVT include unilateral calf or thigh pain, leg swelling, or redness, while symptoms of PE include dyspnea and pleuritic chest pain.[7] Definitive diagnosis of VTE requires radiological imaging, which includes compression ultrasonography (CUS), computed tomography (CT), and conventional venography for DVT and CT pulmonary angiography (CTPA), nuclear medicine lung scintigraphy, and conventional pulmonary angiography for PE.[7,8,9,10]

Treatment of VTE has evolved significantly over time and seeks to prevent propagation of thrombus and long-term recurrent events and address any clinical symptoms in the short term. Early attempts to prevent VTE date back to the late 1800s, when K.G. Lennander, a Swedish surgeon, identified the benefit of hydration to encourage blood circulation as well as compression and elevation of the leg to prevent DVT.[11] In 1937, heparin became available to prevent thrombosis after heart surgery and in 1959, the first controlled trial on the prevention of VTE was published evaluating phenindione, a vitamin K antagonist (VKA), as an effective preventative agent of thrombosis.[11] Starting in the 1970s, clinical trials with low-dose heparin showed its efficacy at preventing DVT in surgical patients.[12] Low-molecular-weight heparin (LMWH) was later evaluated in 1982 due to its longer half-life, improved subcutaneous absorption, and decreased affinity for plasma proteins and platelets compared to unfractionated heparin allowing for longer injection intervals.[13] Once daily injection of LMWH followed by long-term VKA treatment using

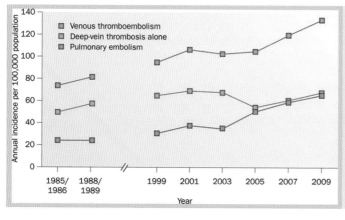

Fig. 1.1 Trend in venous thromboembolism (VTE) incidence over time in the Worcester VTE study from 1985 to 2009. Reproduced with permission from: Huang W, Goldberg RJ, Anderson FA, Kiefe CI, Spencer FA. Secular trends in occurrence of acute venous thromboembolism: the Worcester VTE study (1985–2009). Am J Med 2014;127(9):829–839.

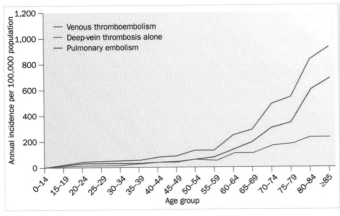

Fig. 1.2 Incidence of venous thromboembolism (VTE) by age from 1966 to 1990 in Olmsted County, MN. Reproduced with permission from: Huang W, Goldberg RJ, Anderson FA, Kiefe CI, Spencer FA. Secular trends in occurrence of acute venous thromboembolism: the Worcester VTE study (1985–2009). Am J Med 2014;127(9):829–839.

warfarin still remains a common modality for preventing VTE in many surgical and medical patients.[11,14] In recent decades, direct oral anticoagulants (DOACs) have become available after extensive clinical trials for the prevention of VTE and are now recommended by the 2016 American College of Chest Physicians and the 2017 European Society of Cardiology guidelines.[15,16] Compared to VKAs, DOACs have a rapid onset of action and more predictable pharmacokinetic profile, which make for simple drug administration without laboratory monitoring or adjustments.[17] DOACs were also identified to be noninferior to LMWH followed by long-term VKA treatment, and were associated with a lower risk of bleeding.[11,15] However, DOACs are avoided in certain patients due to renal impairment, drug–drug interactions, and cost.[17]

Although anticoagulation is the main treatment of VTE, filter placement, thrombolytic therapy, and mechanical interventions to dissolve or remove VTE are also available and commonly used to treat submassive and massive PE.[15,16,18] The first inferior vena cava (IVC) filter was introduced in the late 1960s made to be implanted in the IVC to prevent thrombi from reaching pulmonary circulation.[19] Since their inception, many different types of filters have continued to be developed to reduce complications such as vena cava perforation, filter dislocation, migration, rupture, recurrent VTE, thrombophlebitis, and venous stasis disease.[19] In the late 1970s, streptokinase and urokinase were approved for thrombolytic therapy for acute PE.[20] Thrombolytic therapy involves the use of medication administered systemically or locally, sometimes using catheter-directed therapy (CDT) if systemic therapy is contraindicated due to high

risk of bleeding.[17,21] Tissue plasminogen activator (tPA), which was approved in 1987, is most commonly used today.[22] Historically, thrombolytic therapy was the first-line treatment for only high-risk PE but was then expanded to include treatment for some intermediate-risk PE due to improved outcomes compared to anticoagulant therapy.[15,23] More recently, endovascular techniques have been used in conjunction with local administration of half-dose tPA using CDT to assist in dissolving the thrombus and have evolved over time.[21] Previously, mechanical techniques were only considered in patients who did not qualify for thrombolytic therapy; however, today these techniques are more commonly used as primary reperfusion strategies.[24] The simplest mechanical technique, referred to as fragmentation and published in 2000, involves using a pigtail catheter to fragment the thrombus through repetitive manual rotation of the catheter.[25] More advanced techniques are classified by their mechanism under rheolytic, aspiration, and rotational thrombectomy and will be described in greater detail in later chapters.[21]

Identifying the best therapeutic approach for a patient with VTE is important and often not clear to the practitioner despite extensive guidelines and many new therapeutic options. Understanding the patient's specific clinical circumstances and characteristics is important to identifying an appropriate treatment. For this reason, PE response teams (PERTs) have become more commonplace, bringing a multidisciplinary team together to identify the best management plan using available clinical data and local resources.[26] PERTs allow for the most up-to-date decision-making and have been shown to reduce in-hospital mortality and length of stay, making them an important tool in managing PE.[26] In this textbook, the evaluation and diagnosis of the VTE patient will be described in detail, including medical and interventional therapies currently available and those being developed.

References

[1] Beckman MG, Hooper WC, Critchley SE, Ortel TL. Venous thromboembolism: a public health concern. Am J Prev Med. 2010; 38(4) Suppl:S495–S501

[2] Silverstein MD, Heit JA, Mohr DN, Petterson TM, O'Fallon WM, Melton LJ, III. Trends in the incidence of deep vein thrombosis and pulmonary embolism: a 25-year population-based study. Arch Intern Med. 1998; 158(6):585–593

[3] Spencer FA, Emery C, Lessard D, et al. The Worcester venous thromboembolism study: a population-based study of the clinical epidemiology of venous thromboembolism. J Gen Intern Med. 2006; 21(7):722–727

[4] White RH, Zhou H, Murin S, Harvey D. Effect of ethnicity and gender on the incidence of venous thromboembolism in a diverse population in California in 1996. Thromb Haemost. 2005; 93(2):298–305

[5] Spyropoulos AC, Lin J. Direct medical costs of venous thromboembolism and subsequent hospital readmission rates: an administrative claims analysis from 30 managed care organizations. J Manag Care Pharm. 2007; 13(6):475–486

[6] Preventing Hospital-Associated Venous Thromboembolism. Accessed October 6, 2022 at: https://www.ahrq.gov/patient-safety/settings/hospital/vtguide/index.html

[7] Wells P, Anderson D. The diagnosis and treatment of venous thromboembolism. Hematology (Am Soc Hematol Educ Program). 2013; 2013(1):457–463

[8] Stevens H, McFadyen J, Chan N. Advances in the management of acute venous thromboembolism and new therapeutic agents. Semin Respir Crit Care Med. 2021; 42(2):218–232

[9] Silickas J, Black SA, Phinikaridou A, Gwozdz AM, Smith A, Saha P. Use of computed tomography and magnetic resonance imaging in central venous disease. Methodist DeBakey Cardiovasc J. 2018; 14(3):188–195

[10] Moore AJE, Wachsmann J, Chamarthy MR, Panjikaran L, Tanabe Y, Rajiah P. Imaging of acute pulmonary embolism: an update. Cardiovasc Diagn Ther. 2018; 8(3):225–243

[11] Schulman S, Kearon C, Subcommittee on Control of Anticoagulation of the Scientific and Standardization Committee of the International Society on Thrombosis and Haemostasis. Definition of major bleeding in clinical investigations of antihemostatic medicinal products in non-surgical patients. J Thromb Haemost. 2005; 3(4):692–694

[12] Kakkar VV, Field ES, Nicolaides AN, Flute PT, Wessler S, Yin ET. Low doses of heparin in prevention of deep-vein thrombosis. Lancet. 1971; 2(7726):669–671

[13] Kakkar VV, Djazaeri B, Fok J, Fletcher M, Scully MF, Westwick J. Low-molecular-weight heparin and prevention of postoperative deep vein thrombosis. Br Med J (Clin Res Ed). 1982; 284(6313):375–379

[14] Chan NC, Weitz JI. Recent advances in understanding, diagnosing and treating venous thrombosis. F1000 Research. 2020; 9(1206):1–15

[15] Kearon C, Akl EA, Ornelas J, et al. Antithrombotic therapy for VTE disease: CHEST Guideline and Expert Panel Report. Chest. 2016; 149(2):315–352

[16] Mazzolai L, Aboyans V, Ageno W, et al. Diagnosis and management of acute deep vein thrombosis: a joint consensus document from the European Society of Cardiology working groups of aorta and peripheral vascular diseases and pulmonary circulation and right ventricular function. Eur Heart J. 2018; 39(47):4208–4218

[17] Tritschler T, Kraaijpoel N, Le Gal G, Wells PS. Venous thromboembolism: advances in diagnosis and treatment. JAMA. 2018; 320(15):1583–1594

[18] Hao Q, Dong BR, Yue J, Wu T, Liu GJ. Thrombolytic therapy for pulmonary embolism. Cochrane Database Syst Rev. 2018; 12 (12):CD004437

[19] Ni H, Win LL. Retrievable inferior vena cava filters for venous thromboembolism. ISRN Radiol. 2013; 2013:959452

[20] Dalen JE, Alpert JS, Hirsh J. Thrombolytic therapy for pulmonary embolism: is it effective? Is it safe? When is it indicated? Arch Intern Med. 1997; 157(22):2550–2556

[21] De Gregorio MA, Guirola JA, Lahuerta C, Serrano C, Figueredo AL, Kuo WT. Interventional radiology treatment for pulmonary embolism. World J Radiol. 2017; 9(7):295–303

[22] FDA. ACTIVASE (alteplase) for injection. 1–17. https://www.accessdata.fda.gov/drugsatfda_docs/label/2015/103172s5203lbl.pdf. Published 2015

[23] Chatterjee S, Chakraborty A, Weinberg I, et al. Thrombolysis for pulmonary embolism and risk of all-cause mortality, major bleeding, and intracranial hemorrhage: a meta-analysis. JAMA. 2014; 311(23):2414–2421

[24] Tice C, Seigerman M, Fiorilli P, et al. Management of acute pulmonary embolism. Curr Cardiovasc Risk Rep. 2020; 14 (12):24

[25] Schmitz-Rode T, Janssens U, Duda SH, Erley CM, Günther RW. Massive pulmonary embolism: percutaneous emergency treatment by pigtail rotation catheter. J Am Coll Cardiol. 2000; 36(2):375–380

[26] Annabathula R, Dugan A, Bhalla V, Davis GA, Smyth SS, Gupta VA. Value-based assessment of implementing a Pulmonary Embolism Response Team (PERT). J Thromb Thrombolysis. 2021; 51(1):217–225

Chapter 2

Pharmacologic Management of Venous Thromboembolism

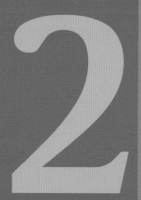

2 Pharmacologic Management of Venous Thromboembolism

Brian J. Carney and Kenneth A. Bauer

Keywords: pharmacology, anticoagulation, thrombolytics

2.1 Role of Pharmacologic Treatment of VTE

Pharmacologic treatment is central to the management of deep vein thrombosis (DVT) and pulmonary embolism (PE). Commonly used agents include systemic thrombolytics for massive PE and, more commonly, anticoagulants such as heparin and heparin derivatives, warfarin, and several newer oral agents. The role of anticoagulant therapy in DVT and PE is to stabilize existing thrombi, prevent the formation of new thrombi, and thereby allow for endogenous fibrinolysis to break down thrombi. Anticoagulants do not have intrinsic "clot busting" activity as do plasminogen activators such as tissue plasminogen activator (tPA). This chapter will focus on the management of venous thromboembolism (VTE) with anticoagulants. For an overview of thrombolysis, please see Chapter 9.

Long-term management of DVT and PE is driven largely by whether the index clot(s) was *provoked* or *unprovoked*. A provoked clot is one that occurs in the setting of a recognized risk factor for venous thrombosis. Provoking factors may be temporary, such as major surgery, admission to the hospital for greater than 3 days, estrogen therapy, pregnancy and puerperium, and lower extremity injury associated with reduced mobility for at least 3 days. Provoking factors may also be persistent, such as active malignancy or conditions causing chronic systemic inflammation (e.g., inflammatory bowel disease).[1] An unprovoked DVT or PE is one that occurs in the absence of obvious risk factors. Anticoagulation for 3 to 6 months is typically sufficient for a DVT or PE occurring in the setting of a temporary provoking factor. Indefinite anticoagulation is commonly recommended for patients with a persistent risk factor and in those with truly unprovoked clots. For an in-depth overview of current recommendations regarding choice and duration of anticoagulation for DVT and PE, please see the most recent American College of Chest Physicians (ACCP) guidelines on VTE.[2]

2.2 Traditional Anticoagulants

2.2.1 Heparins and Heparin Derivatives

Heparin is a naturally occurring glycosaminoglycan that is produced by mast cells and basophils. The physiologic role of heparin is incompletely understood. As an anticoagulant, it is commonly given as unfractionated heparin, which consists of a mixture of polysaccharides with a mean chain length of 45 saccharide units. The mechanism of action of heparin is primarily mediated by its binding to antithrombin (AT). In doing so, heparin induces a conformational change in AT that potentiates its inhibition of both thrombin and factor Xa.

Dosing of heparin is weight-based. For acute DVT and PE, heparin is usually initiated with an intravenous (IV) bolus of either 80 units/kg or 5,000 units total. Subsequently, heparin is given via a continuous IV infusion at either 18 units/kg/hour or 1,000 units/hour.[3] In terms of monitoring and dose adjustment, anticoagulation to an activated partial thromboplastin time (aPTT) of between 1.5 and 2.5 times the institutional upper limit of normal (usually 60–80 seconds) is targeted. When the aPTT is outside of this range, dose adjustment, bolus, and/or temporary holding of heparin may be appropriate. An example of a typical heparin nomogram is shown in ▶ Table 2.1. No dose adjustment is needed for renal or hepatic dysfunction; monitoring and titration are as per the aPTT as described above.

Another commonly prescribed form of heparin is low-molecular weight heparin (LMWH), which is derived by isolating lower molecular weight fragments from heparin, thereby producing a fractionated mixture. The mean length of LMWH fragments is 15 saccharide units. Mechanistically, LMWH is similar to heparin in that it binds to AT resulting in a conformational change that potentiates inhibition of factor Xa. Unlike heparin, LMWH affects the activity of thrombin to a lesser extent than factor Xa. Dosing of LMWH is straightforward; see ▶ Table 2.2 for initial dosing schemes for several Food and Drug Administration (FDA)-approved agents. LMWHs, particularly enoxaparin, have an increased half-life in patients with renal

Table 2.1 Typical heparin nomogram

aPTT	Bolus (units)	Hold (minutes)	Rate change (units/hour)
0–39.9	5,000	-	Increase infusion rate by 400 units/hour
40–59.9	2,500	-	Increase infusion rate by 200 units/hour
60–99.9	-	-	None
100–119.9	-	-	Reduce infusion rate by 200 units/hour
>120	-	60	Reduce infusion rate by 400 units/hour

Abbreviation: aPTT, activated partial thromboplastin time.

Table 2.2 Low-molecular weight heparin initial dosing schemes

LMWH	Dosing for acute VTE
Dalteparin	200 units/kg once daily
Enoxaparin	1 mg/kg Q12 H or 1.5 mg/kg once daily
Nadroparin	171 units/kg once daily
Tinzaparin	175 units/kg once daily

Abbreviations: LMWH, low-molecular weight heparin; VTE, venous thromboembolism.

failure, especially with a creatinine clearance of less than 30 mL/minute, and therefore must be used with caution in this population. It is not always necessary to monitor LMWH therapy; however, when desired, this can be accomplished by using a chromogenic anti-factor Xa assay.

As with any anticoagulant medication, one of the most common adverse effects of heparin or LMWH therapy is bleeding. This can range from self-limited mucocutaneous bleeding to major and potentially fatal hemorrhage. The management of minor bleeding with heparin is usually a combination of local measures and holding of the drug. In the event of more serious bleeding (e.g., intracranial hemorrhage), reversal is indicated. Protamine sulfate is approved for the reversal of heparin; it partially neutralizes the anticoagulant activity of LMWH. It accomplishes this through ionic association with the heparin polysaccharide, thereby eliminating its anticoagulant activity. To reverse unfractionated heparin, protamine sulfate can be given at a dose of 1 mg for every 100 units of heparin administered during the preceding 30 to 60 minutes. Alternatively, a single dose of 25 or 50 mg can be given. Reversal of LMWH is dependent on the particular formulation used. For details on the reversal of LMWH, please consult local pharmacy guidelines.

Other than bleeding, one of the most common adverse effects of heparin and LMWH is heparin-induced thrombocytopenia (HIT). HIT is an immunologic disorder driven by the development of platelet-activating antibodies against an epitope of platelet factor 4 (PF4) associated with the heparin polysaccharide. HIT is common in hospitalized patients receiving therapeutic and prophylactic doses of heparin, occurring at a rate of up to 1 in 5,000. Clinically, HIT is characterized by a fall in the platelet count of greater than 50% in 5 to 10 days after initiating a heparin product. Despite thrombocytopenia, HIT is associated with a markedly hypercoagulable state with risk of both arterial and venous thrombosis. In a patient with a decrease in platelet count while on heparin, the 4T score (► Table 2.3) can be used to determine the pre-test probability of HIT and appropriateness of additional laboratory testing and possibly treatment.[4] A 4T score of four or higher warrants testing for antibodies against the PF4-heparin polysaccharide epitope, also known as heparin-dependent antibodies. A decidedly positive heparin-dependent antibody is an indication for treatment of HIT. An equivocal result may necessitate confirmatory testing with a serotonin release assay.

Treatment of laboratory-confirmed HIT begins with holding of all heparin products. As HIT carries a significant risk of thrombosis, immediate reinstitution of anticoagulation with a nonheparin agent is mandatory. Agents used for anticoagulation in the setting of HIT include parenteral direct-thrombin inhibitors argatroban and bivalirudin. Clearance of argatroban is primarily hepatic, and as such bivalirudin is preferred in the setting of liver dysfunction. There is a growing body of evidence supporting the use of

Table 2.3 4 T score

	Score = 2	Score = 1	Score = 0
Thrombocytopenia	Platelet count falls > 50% *and* platelet nadir > 20 K/μL	Platelet count falls 30–50% *or* platelet nadir 10–19 K/μL	Platelet count falls < 30% *or* platelet nadir < 10 K/μL
Timing of fall in platelet count	Clear onset between days 5 and 10 of heparin exposure *or* platelet count falls at ≤ 1 day with prior heparin exposure within 30 days	Consistent with fall in platelet count at 5–10 days, but not clear (e.g., missing platelet counts) *or* onset after day 10 *or* falls ≤ 1 day with prior heparin exposure 30–100 days ago	Platelet count falls in < 4 days without prior heparin exposure in past 100 days
Thrombosis	New thrombosis, skin necrosis at heparin injection site, anaphylactoid reaction after intravenous (IV) unfractionated heparin bolus	Progressive or recurrent thrombosis, nonnecrotizing (erythematous) skin lesions, suspected thrombosis	None evident
Other causes of thrombocytopenia	None evident	Possible	Definite (e.g., sepsis or severe infection, disseminated intravascular coagulation (DIC), new medication known to cause thrombocytopenia)

fondaparinux, a synthetic heparin derivative containing only the pentasaccharide fragment, for HIT. Fondaparinux does not form aggregates with PF4 and thus lacks the potential of larger polysaccharide fragments for inducing HIT. Rivaroxaban and apixaban, both oral factor Xa inhibitors, are being studied for the treatment of HIT. For further discussion of rivaroxaban and apixaban and other newer anticoagulants, please see later in this chapter. For a more in-depth discussion of HIT, please see the excellent review by Greinacher.[5]

2.2.2 Warfarin

The anticoagulant effect of warfarin is mediated by its inhibition of the vitamin K-dependent synthesis of a number of coagulation factors, specifically factors II, VII, IX, and X; it also decreases the synthesis of the endogenous anticoagulants, proteins C and S. Warfarin inhibits the VKORC1 subunit of vitamin K epoxide reductase, thereby decreasing the availability of reduced vitamin K to participate in the synthesis of the above coagulation factors. For the treatment of VTE, initiation of warfarin requires "bridging" or concomitant administration of heparin. The reason for this is two-fold. First, warfarin takes several days to achieve a therapeutic effect, during which time heparin provides the

needed systemic anticoagulation. Second, levels of endogenous anticoagulants proteins C and S fall more rapidly than several vitamin K-dependent coagulation factors (i.e., prothrombin, factor IX, and factor X) following the initiation of warfarin, thus creating the potential for an increased risk of thrombosis. For these reasons, combined therapy with heparin and warfarin should be overlapped for at least 5 days. Prior to stopping heparin, warfarin should be therapeutic for at least 24 hours. Initial dosing of warfarin is patient-specific, although starting doses of 5 to 10 mg are typical.

Warfarin is monitored using the prothrombin time (PT) from which the international normalized ratio (INR) is derived. Dosing is usually adjusted to an INR of 2 to 3, although a higher target is occasionally used for patients with recurrent thrombosis while on therapeutic anticoagulation and for markedly thrombophilic states such as high-risk antiphospholipid antibody syndrome; an INR target range of 2.5 to 3.5 is recommended for patients with mechanical heart valves. The management of warfarin is complicated given a number of drug–drug interactions (▶ Table 2.4) and susceptibility of the INR to abrupt dietary changes. For example, an abrupt increase in dietary vitamin K intake (e.g., spinach) could blunt the pharmacologic effect of warfarin resulting in an INR below goal. Despite

Table 2.4 Common drug–drug interactions with warfarin

Increase INR	Decrease INR
Amiodarone	Barbiturates
Azole antifungals	Carbamazepine
Cimetidine	Cholestyramine
Fluoroquinolone antibiotics	Estrogens
Fluorouracil	Phenytoin
Levothyroxine	Rifampin
Macrolide antibiotics	Vitamin K
Metronidazole	
Proton pump inhibitors	
Trimethoprim-sulfamethoxazole. (TMP-SMX)	

Abbreviation: INR, international normalized ratio.

this, patients starting warfarin should *not* be advised to avoid foods that are high in vitamin K, many of which are quite nutritious. Rather, they should be encouraged to maintain a consistent vitamin K intake so as to allow for stable warfarin dosing.

As with heparin and LMWHs, warfarin occasionally requires reversal in the setting of active bleeding or should a need for an urgent surgical procedure arise. Nonurgent reversal can be accomplished by holding warfarin and allowing the INR to gradually decrease over a period of several days. Alternatively, this process could be expedited with doses of IV, oral, or subcutaneous vitamin K; IV administration results in the most rapid correction of the INR. When more urgent reversal is indicated, one of the most commonly employed strategies is infusion of fresh frozen plasma (FFP), which is a whole blood-derived product containing all endogenous coagulation factors. Alternatively, major bleeding with warfarin can be managed with a prothrombin complex concentrate (PCC), which contains factors VII, II, IX, and X; the four-factor PCC presently available in the United States is commercially known as Kcentra. There are limited data comparing the efficacy of FFP to PCC. A meta-analysis of several large retrospective studies was suggestive of superiority of PCC in terms of all-cause mortality[6]; however, a recent randomized controlled trial in patients with intracranial hemorrhage on a vitamin K antagonist failed to demonstrate a convincing clinical benefit of PCC relative to FFP beyond more rapid INR correction.[7]

2.3 Newer Anticoagulants

Rivaroxaban, apixaban, and edoxaban are oral factor Xa inhibitors. Dabigatran is an oral direct thrombin inhibitor. Unlike warfarin, these agents do not require laboratory monitoring, have few drug–drug interactions, and their anticoagulant effect is not impacted by diet. The following paragraphs will review the registration studies that led to the FDA approval of rivaroxaban, apixaban, edoxaban, and dabigatran for acute VTE.

Rivaroxaban was evaluated for symptomatic DVT in the 2010 EINSTEIN-DVT study and for PE in the 2012 EINSTEIN-PE study. In EINSTEIN-DVT and EINSTEIN-PE studies, patients with proximal DVT or PE were randomized to either rivaroxaban or enoxaparin followed by warfarin with a goal INR of 2 to 3. In both the trials, rivaroxaban was given without initial parenteral anticoagulation and administered at a dose of 15 mg twice daily for 21 days followed by 20 mg once daily for the remainder of the study period. Rivaroxaban was found to be noninferior to warfarin in terms of rates of recurrent VTE in both EINSTEIN-DVT and EINSTEIN-PE. There was no significant difference in terms of bleeding risk in either study.[8,9] On the basis of these data, rivaroxaban was approved for the treatment of acute VTE in July 2011.

Apixaban was evaluated for use in acute VTE in the 2013 AMPLIFY study, in which 5,395 patients with proximal DVT or PE were randomized to receive either apixaban or enoxaparin followed by warfarin with a goal INR of 2 to 3. Apixaban was given without initial parenteral anticoagulation and administered at a dose of 10 mg twice daily for 7 days followed by 5 mg twice daily for 6 months. At 6 months follow-up, apixaban was found to be noninferior to conventional therapy in terms of preventing recurrent VTE and in VTE-related death. Additionally, apixaban was associated with significantly fewer episodes of major and nonmajor bleeding.[10] On the basis of these data, apixaban was approved for the treatment of acute VTE in March 2014.

Edoxaban was evaluated for use in acute VTE in the 2013 Hokusai VTE study, in which 4,921 patients with acute VTE were randomized to receive either edoxaban 60 mg once daily or warfarin with a goal INR of 2 to 3. Dose reductions in edoxaban to 30 mg once daily were allowed in patients with a creatinine clearance of 30 to 50 mL/minute, a body weight of 60 kg or less, and in patients who were receiving concomitant treatment with a potent P-glycoprotein inhibitor. Notably, unlike in the registration studies for rivaroxaban and apixaban, edoxaban was initiated following a parenteral anticoagulant, most commonly unfractionated or LMWH, which was given for the first 5 days of VTE therapy. At 6 months follow-up, rates of recurrent VTE were similar between the edoxaban and warfarin arms. Edoxaban was associated with significantly fewer episodes of major and clinically relevant nonmajor bleeding.[11] On the basis of these data, edoxaban was approved for the treatment of acute VTE in January 2015.

The 2009 RE-COVER study investigated the use of dabigatran for acute VTE. In total, 2,500 patients with DVT and PE were randomized to receive dabigatran 150 mg twice daily or dose-adjusted warfarin. Similar to the Hokusai VTE study, dabigatran was initiated following a parenteral anticoagulant, most commonly unfractionated or LMWH, which was given for the first 5 days of VTE therapy. At 6 months follow-up, rates of recurrent VTE and VTE-related death were similar between the dabigatran and conventional therapy arms. There was no difference in major bleeding; however, there were significantly fewer episodes of total bleeding with dabigatran.[12] On the basis of these data, dabigatran gained FDA approval for acute VTE in April 2014.

In summary, rivaroxaban, apixaban, edoxaban, and dabigatran, which are often collectively referred to as direct oral anticoagulants or "DOACs,"

are at least as effective and safe as warfarin for the management of acute DVT and PE. Given this and the added convenience for both patients and providers, DOACs are now considered first-line therapy for VTE in patients without cancer as per the most recent ACCP guidelines on VTE.[2] A summary of the accepted initiation and dosing schemes of DOACs is provided in ▶ Table 2.5.

When initially approved by the FDA, none of the DOACs had an available reversal agent. The first such agent developed was idarucizumab, a humanized antibody fragment that binds with high affinity to dabigatran and its metabolites, thereby reversing its anticoagulant effect. Idarucizumab was evaluated in the single-arm REVERSE-AD study, in which patients with major bleeding or requiring operative procedures on dabigatran were rapidly administered 5 mg of the drug intravenously (i.e., two 2.5 mg vials). This treatment resulted in 100% reversal of the dabigatran anticoagulant effect by 4 hours post-infusion. Clinically, bleeding patients were observed to achieve hemostasis at a median of 11.4 hours and 33/35 of patients requiring surgery had acceptable intraoperative hemostasis as judged by the treating clinicians. Five thrombotic events occurred in REVERSE-AD, one within 72 hours of idarucizumab infusion and four at a later time. Notably, none of these five patients were on antithrombotic therapy at the time of thrombosis.[13] On the basis of REVERSE-AD data, idarucizumab was approved by the FDA in October 2015.

Andexanet alfa is a recombinant, genetically engineered version of human factor Xa that has high affinity for factor Xa inhibitors such as LMWH, rivaroxaban, apixaban, and edoxaban; it interacts minimally with other coagulation and regulatory proteins. Andexanet alfa was evaluated for acute major bleeding in patients on these medications in the ANNEXA-4 study. Patients with bleeding on

Table 2.5 DOACs

DOAC	Initial parenteral anticoagulation	Initial dosing	Subsequent dosing
Apixaban	None	10 mg twice daily for 7 days	5 mg twice daily
Rivaroxaban	None	15 mg twice daily for 21 days	20 mg once daily
Edoxaban	5–10 days	-	60 mg once daily
Dabigatran	5–10 days	-	150 mg twice daily

Abbreviation: DOACs, direct oral anticoagulants.

rivaroxaban or apixaban were treated with an initial bolus and then a 2-hour infusion of andexanet alfa. This resulted in an 89 to 93% reduction in the anticoagulant effect of these drugs, and 31 out of 47 patients achieved hemostasis that was judged as normal. Thrombotic events occurred in 12 out of 67 patients who were evaluated in the safety population.[14] On the basis of these data, andexanet alfa was approved by the FDA in May 2018.

There are a number of additional cautions with DOACs that warrant discussion. Interactions with other drugs, while substantially less common than with warfarin, can occur. Medications that strongly induce CYP3A4, for example, rifampicin and several antiepileptics, lead to more rapid DOAC metabolism and thus a blunted anticoagulant effect. Patients with significant chronic kidney disease or end-stage renal disease, morbid obesity, and altered gastrointestinal anatomy (e.g., gastric bypass) were not included in large numbers in any of the registration trials described above; therefore, DOACs should be used with greater caution in these populations. There are no data as to whether DOACs are safe during pregnancy or the postpartum period, and because of this, they should be avoided in women who are pregnant and those planning to breastfeed.

2.4 Special Populations

There are several special populations that warrant discussion. Patients with active malignancy are at an increased risk for VTE. Historically, LMWH has been the standard of care for cancer-associated thrombosis on the basis of the CLOT study, in which LMWH was shown to be superior to warfarin in preventing recurrent VTE without added risk of bleeding.[15] In the more recent Hokusai VTE cancer study, edoxaban was compared to LMWH. Edoxaban was found to be noninferior to LMWH in terms of a composite outcome of recurrent VTE or major bleeding. Notably, the rate of recurrent VTE was lower in the edoxaban arm while the rate of major bleeding was higher, particularly in patients with gastrointestinal malignancies.[16] Clinical trials assessing the safety and efficacy of other DOACs in patients with active malignancy are ongoing.

Antiphospholipid antibody syndrome (APLS) is an autoimmune disorder characterized by increased risk of both venous and arterial thrombosis. VTE occurring in the setting of APLS should be managed with heparin or LMWH followed by warfarin with a goal INR of 2 to 3. Recently, several groups have

sought to assess the safety and efficacy of DOACs for APLS-associated VTE. One of the largest clinical trials in this area was the TRAPS study, in which patients with high-risk APLS, defined as positivity for lupus anticoagulant, beta-2 glycoprotein I antibodies, and cardiolipin antibodies, with history of thrombosis were randomized to receive either rivaroxaban or warfarin. The TRAPS study was terminated prematurely, after enrollment of only 120 patients, due to an excess number of thrombotic events with rivaroxaban.[17] Although these data raise concerns regarding the efficacy of DOACs in APLS, it is important to note that this was a population at a particularly high risk of recurrent thrombosis. Further studies seeking to assess the efficacy of DOACs in lower-risk APLS populations are ongoing.

There are a number of hereditary thrombophilias that may be identified after a first venous thrombotic event. These include but are not limited to mutations in the genes encoding Factor V (Leiden) and prothrombin (G20210A mutation) and deficiencies in endogenous anticoagulants such as AT and proteins C and S. At the time of this writing, there is no evidence to suggest that any of the above anticoagulants are more or less effective for patients with hereditary thrombophilias than warfarin.

References

[1] Kearon C, Ageno W, Cannegieter SC, Cosmi B, Geersing GJ, Kyrle PA, Subcommittees on Control of Anticoagulation, and Predictive and Diagnostic Variables in Thrombotic Disease. Categorization of patients as having provoked or unprovoked venous thromboembolism: guidance from the SSC of ISTH. J Thromb Haemost. 2016; 14(7):1480–1483

[2] Kearon C, Akl EA, Ornelas J, et al. Antithrombotic therapy for VTE disease: CHEST guideline and expert panel report. Chest. 2016; 149(2):315–352

[3] Holbrook A, Schulman S, Witt DM, et al. Evidence-based management of anticoagulant therapy: Antithrombotic Therapy and Prevention of Thrombosis, 9th ed: American College of Chest Physicians Evidence-Based Clinical Practice Guidelines. Chest. 2012; 141(2) Suppl:e152S–e184S

[4] Lo GK, Juhl D, Warkentin TE, Sigouin CS, Eichler P, Greinacher A. Evaluation of pretest clinical score (4 T's) for the diagnosis of heparin-induced thrombocytopenia in two clinical settings. J Thromb Haemost. 2006; 4(4):759–765

[5] Greinacher A. Heparin-induced thrombocytopenia. N Engl J Med. 2015; 373(19):1883–1884

[6] Chai-Adisaksopha C, Hillis C, Siegal DM, et al. Prothrombin complex concentrates versus fresh frozen plasma for warfarin reversal. A systematic review and meta-analysis. Thromb Haemost. 2016; 116(5):879–890

[7] Steiner T, Poli S, Griebe M, et al. Fresh frozen plasma versus prothrombin complex concentrate in patients with intracranial haemorrhage related to vitamin K antagonists (INCH): a randomised trial. Lancet Neurol. 2016; 15(6):566–573

[8] Bauersachs R, Berkowitz SD, Brenner B, et al. EINSTEIN Investigators. Oral rivaroxaban for symptomatic venous thromboembolism. N Engl J Med. 2010; 363(26):2499–2510

[9] Büller HR, Prins MH, Lensin AW, et al. EINSTEIN–PE Investigators. Oral rivaroxaban for the treatment of symptomatic pulmonary embolism. N Engl J Med. 2012; 366(14):1287–1297

[10] Agnelli G, Buller HR, Cohen A, et al. AMPLIFY Investigators. Oral apixaban for the treatment of acute venous thromboembolism. N Engl J Med. 2013; 369(9):799–808

[11] Büller HR, Décousus H, Grosso MA, et al. Hokusai-VTE Investigators. Edoxaban versus warfarin for the treatment of symptomatic venous thromboembolism. N Engl J Med. 2013; 369(15):1406–1415

[12] Schulman S, Kearon C, Kakkar AK, et al. RE-COVER Study Group. Dabigatran versus warfarin in the treatment of acute venous thromboembolism. N Engl J Med. 2009; 361(24):2342–2352

[13] Pollack CV, Jr, Reilly PA, van Ryn J, et al. Idarucizumab for dabigatran reversal—full cohort analysis. N Engl J Med. 2017; 377(5):431–441

[14] Connolly SJ, Milling TJ, Jr, Eikelboom JW, et al. ANNEXA-4 Investigators. Andexanet alfa for acute major bleeding associated with factor Xa inhibitors. N Engl J Med. 2016; 375(12):1131–1141

[15] Lee AY, Levine MN, Baker RI, et al. Randomized Comparison of Low-Molecular-Weight Heparin versus Oral Anticoagulant Therapy for the Prevention of Recurrent Venous Thromboembolism in Patients with Cancer (CLOT) Investigators. Low-molecular-weight heparin versus a coumarin for the prevention of recurrent venous thromboembolism in patients with cancer. N Engl J Med. 2003; 349(2):146–153

[16] Raskob GE, van Es N, Verhamme P, et al. Hokusai VTE Cancer Investigators. Edoxaban for the treatment of cancer-associated venous thromboembolism. N Engl J Med. 2018; 378(7):615–624

[17] Pengo V, Denas G, Zoppellaro G, et al. Rivaroxaban vs warfarin in high-risk patients with antiphospholipid syndrome. Blood. 2018; 132(13):1365–1371

Chapter 3

Imaging of Deep Vein Thrombosis and Pulmonary Emboli

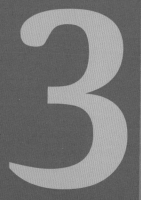

3 Imaging of Deep Vein Thrombosis and Pulmonary Emboli

Olga R. Brook

Keywords: computed tomography, nuclear medicine, lung scan, ultrasound

3.1 Ultrasound

Ultrasound is the imaging modality of choice for diagnosis of deep vein thrombosis (DVT) in the extremities[1] since studies in the early 1980s first showed its value.[2,3] Ultrasound is cost-effective, relatively accurate, portable, and does not require radiation exposure and therefore can be utilized successfully in the variety of health care settings.

3.1.1 Accuracy of Doppler Ultrasound for Diagnosis of DVT

The accuracy of DVT diagnosis with ultrasound varies depending on the presence of symptoms (symptomatic [pain, swelling, and cramping] vs. asymptomatic) and suspected anatomical location of DVT (proximal lower extremity, distal lower extremity, or upper extremity). Asymptomatic DVT is diagnosed when ultrasound is performed for risk stratification in patients with pulmonary emboli (PE) or in screening patients with cancer or immobile patients. Approximately one-third of patients with DVT do not have any symptoms.[4]

Lower extremity: A review of studies and systematic review by Segal et al showed that for *symptomatic* patients, sensitivity of Doppler ultrasound for *proximal lower extremity* thrombosis ranges from 89 to 96% with specificity of 94 to 99%.[5] In different studies, the accuracy of *symptomatic distal lower extremity* DVT ranges from 75 to 93% in sensitivity and from 73 to 99% in specificity.[6,7,8] Sensitivity of detecting DVT in *asymptomatic* patients is significantly lower, ranging from 47 to 62%; however, specificity remains high at 94 to 97%.[8,9]

Upper extremity: Di Nisio et al conducted a systematic review of 11 studies involving symptomatic patients and found that despite the fact that overall most studies suffer from poor methodology, it appears that sensitivities of compression ultrasound with and without Doppler or Doppler

ultrasound by itself or contrast venography are similar, ranging from 85 to 97% with specificity ranging from 87 to 96%, with lower numbers for contrast venography.[10] The authors suggest that the addition of Doppler did not seem to make a significant difference, while the best accuracy is provided by compression ultrasound alone. However, given the overall low quality of available literature, it is prudent to perform compression ultrasound with Doppler to rule out upper extremity DVT (▶ Table 3.1).

3.1.2 Indication

DVT in lower extremities has an estimated incidence of 5/10,000 patients per year in the general population with incidence increasing with age and comorbidities.[11] PE have been diagnosed in up to 60% of patients with DVT, especially as it progresses more centrally from the calf veins. Death

Table 3.1 Summary of accuracy of ultrasound for detection of deep vein thrombosis (DVT)

	Lower extremity	
	Proximal	Distal
Symptomatic	Sensitivity: 89–96% Specificity: 94–96%	Sensitivity: 75–93% Specificity: 73–99%
Asymptomatic	Sensitivity: 47–62% Specificity: 94–97%	
	Upper extremity (symptomatic only)	
Compression ultrasound	Sensitivity: 97% Specificity: 96%	
Doppler ultrasound	Sensitivity: 84% Specificity: 94%	
Compression + Doppler	Sensitivity: 91% Specificity: 93%	
Contrast venography	Sensitivity: 84% Specificity: 87%	

from all causes occurs in approximately 6% of DVT cases and 12% of PE cases within 1 month of diagnosis.[12] Several algorithms have been developed to assess the pretest probability of DVT to accurately detect patients at higher risk of DVT and PE, while reducing unnecessary imaging studies. The Wells criteria, based on clinical signs and symptoms that are most commonly used in clinical practice,[13] classified patients into risk categories for thromboembolic disease as low, intermediate, or high. Patients with low or intermediate risk should be further evaluated with serum D-dimer, while patients classified as high risk should be evaluated with CT pulmonary angiogram to rule out PE. More recently, Le Gal et al simplified risk groups to "DVT likely" and "DVT unlikely."[14] Because the prevalence of DVT in the "DVT unlikely" or low-risk groups is not zero, a follow-up D-dimer test is recommended for further decision-making.[5] If the D-dimer test is negative, a DVT can be safely excluded. If a D-dimer test is positive, patients should undergo ultrasound evaluation of the symptomatic extremity. In a patient with intermediate or high risk or "DVT likely," D-dimer evaluation is unnecessary and ultrasound evaluation will be required to rule out DVT.

3.1.3 Technique

Collaborative practice guidelines for peripheral venous ultrasound examinations were developed by the American College of Radiology, American Institute of Ultrasound in Medicine, Society for Pediatric Radiology, and Society of Radiologists in Ultrasound to set standards for evaluation of venous thromboembolism (VTE) in both the lower and upper extremities.[15] Evaluation of the lower extremity generally begins with optimal grayscale ultrasound technique in both the transverse and sagittal planes, beginning with the common femoral and femoral veins moving down to the popliteal vein, distal to the tibioperoneal trunk. Similarly, evaluation of the upper extremity should include the internal jugular, subclavian, axillary, brachial, cephalic, and basilic veins in both the transverse and sagittal planes. In both examinations, compression by the ultrasound transducer is applied every 2 cm or less in the transverse plane to completely compress the normal vein lumen to eliminate a possibility of acute isoechoic thrombus or lack of thrombus visualization due to poor technique or technical factors. Areas of clinical concern,

such as focal pain, require special attention with focal imaging in the transverse and sagittal planes. Doppler waveforms should be obtained in the bilateral common femoral veins and bilateral subclavian veins, to evaluate for asymmetry or loss of phasicity during the respiratory cycle that will indicate distal (pelvic) thrombus or compression of the pelvic veins. Doppler waveforms should be obtained in the sagittal plane. At the authors' institution, in lower extremity evaluation, compression ultrasound is extended to the posterior tibial veins and peroneal veins. Additionally, augmentation is utilized at our institution at the common femoral, femoral, and popliteal veins when obtaining sagittal Doppler waveforms. Augmentation is a sonographic technique when manual compression or a "squeeze" is briefly applied below the level being imaged (i.e., if imaging the upper calf, transient compression of the lower calf). A brief increase in venous inflow should be visualized on Doppler ultrasound. Lack of increase in venous inflow indicates obstruction to the flow (thrombus or mass) between the area of the "squeeze" and imaging site. Augmentation should be avoided if thrombus is visualized, as it may dislodge the thrombus and cause a pulmonary embolus. Finally, if DVT is identified on a unilateral study, in the authors' institution, the contralateral leg needs are assessed to determine the burden of the disease.

3.1.4 Imaging Features

The imaging features of acute DVT include presence of echogenic clot within a distended and noncompressible vein, without or limited color flow on Doppler imaging. Imaging features that can be seen in chronic DVT include thickened vessel walls, atretic or diminutive venous segments, and the presence of collateral vessels. Chronic clot will become more echogenic over time and can calcify.[16] The clot can have varying degrees of echogenicity, up to being completely anechoic in hyperacute presentation.[16] Therefore, lack of vein compression by the ultrasound transducer is the most definitive test for the detection of DVT. Pelvic DVT can be detected by indirect sonographic signs, such as lack of normal respiratory variation with respiration and Valsalva maneuvers with Doppler tracing over common femoral vein (► Fig. 3.1). Further evaluation with computed tomography (CT) or magnetic resonance (MR) venography can be useful in this scenario.[17] Indirect signs of DVT in the calf veins

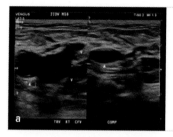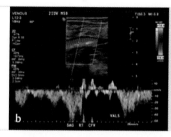

Fig. 3.1 (a) Normal transverse images of the right common femoral vein (CFV) with and without compression. (b) Normal color Doppler and waveform in the right CFV showing normal respiratory variation and Valsalva.

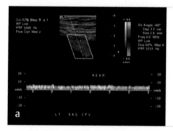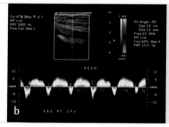

Fig. 3.2 (a) Abnormal respiration variability of the left common femoral vein (CFV) raising suspicion for distal (central) pathology. Confirmed left deep venous thrombosis in a case of May–Thurner syndrome. (b) The same patient with normal right CFV respiration variability.

are lack of augmentation (increase in flow) with calf squeeze in the deep thigh veins as seen on Doppler ultrasound[16] (▶ Fig. 3.2).

3.1.5 Pitfalls

False-positive ultrasound diagnosis of DVT can be caused by pelvic masses compressing vasculature, such as adenopathy, malignancy, abscesses, and hematomas, as well as diffuse soft-tissue edema. At times, an arterial abnormality can be confused for venous one.[16]

Important pitfall for false-negative results is aberrant anatomy, such as duplicated femoral and popliteal veins. In these cases, all veins should be evaluated for DVT.[17] *Patient factors*, such as morbid obesity, extreme edema, postoperative bandaging, and lack of cooperation with the sonographer can also limit usefulness of the study.

Technical expertise of the sonographer as well as use of the established protocol is of vast importance in reducing variability and thus improving accuracy of the examination.

3.2 Computed Tomography Pulmonary Angiography

Use of computed tomography pulmonary angiography (CTPA) for diagnosis of PE has increased significantly since 1992, when it was shown to be as effective as conventional angiography[18] and

more accurate than ventilation perfusion (V/Q) scan. Multidetector CTPA has been shown to have a sensitivity of 83% and specificity of 96%, as identified in the Prospective Investigation of Pulmonary Embolism Diagnosis (PIOPED) II study.[19]

3.2.1 Indication

Evaluation of a patient's pretest probability of pulmonary embolism can be performed using several decision-making tools, including Wells' criteria, Geneva criteria, and pulmonary embolism rule-out criteria (PERC).[20,21,22] Using these tools, low- and intermediate-risk patients undergo high-sensitivity D-dimer testing. A negative D-dimer effectively excludes deep venous thrombosis.[23] In intermediate-risk patients with a positive D-dimer or those with a high pretest probability of pulmonary embolism, multidetector CTPA is indicated.[24,25]

3.2.2 Technique

The CTPA technique has continued to evolve over time with the improving technology of CT scanners, although the main premise behind the examination has not significantly changed. Axial CT imaging is obtained from the lung apices to the diaphragm following administration of intravenous (IV) contrast, with the scan timed for opacification of the pulmonary arteries. Optimally, CTPA is obtained using 16- or 64-channel multidetector CT scanner to allow for single breath hold imaging to

BMI	kVp	IV contrast (cc)	LA threshold (HU)
<25	80	80	170
25-33	100	100	135
>35	120	120	100

Fig. 3.3 kVp, contrast dose, and scan triggering threshold based on the patient's body mass index (BMI).

reduce motion artifacts. In our institution, kVp, volume of contrast, and HU threshold for scan initiation are chosen based on the patient's body mass index (BMI; ▶ Fig. 3.3) in order to improve vessel opacification while reducing radiation exposure and contrast load. A bolus tracking technique is recommended for optimal timing of the scan, usually focused on the main pulmonary artery. At the authors' institution, the left atrium is used to track the bolus with the scan obtained during shallow inspiration in order to perform "a double rule-out" to evaluate for both PE and aortic dissection, as symptoms between these conditions can sometimes overlap. Scan slices are acquired in thin 0.5-mm sections, with 2.5- and 1.25-mm axial reformats produced for review. In addition, 5-mm sagittal and coronal and 15-mm maximal intensity projections (MIPs) of left and right oblique images are obtained to demonstrate pulmonary vasculature. Our protocol allows for opacification of both pulmonary arterial and central arterial circulation in order to rule out both PE and aortic dissection. This "double rule-out" technique requires larger volume contrast than solely targeting pulmonary circulation, which can be performed with as little as 40 mL of IV contrast with concentration of 350 to 370 mgI/mL (milligrams of iodine/milliliter) and utilization of low kVp in patients with small body habitus.

3.2.3 Imaging Features

Diagnosis of pulmonary embolism on CTPA is made by identification of filling defects in the pulmonary arteries. The filling defect may cause a complete occlusion of the vessel with nonenhancing vessel, a

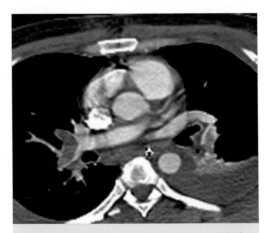

Fig. 3.4 Filling defect in the distal right main and left lower lobar pulmonary arteries.

partial central filling defect, or a peripheral filling defect (▶ Fig. 3.4).[26] A complete filling defect may also result in vessel enlargement compared to adjacent or contralateral, nonoccluded pulmonary arteries. In the case of a partial filling defect, the "polo mint" sign may be seen on transverse slices through a vessel with central hypoattenuation surrounded by hyperattenuating contrast material (▶ Fig. 3.5). Longitudinal slices through the vessel will demonstrate a "tram track" sign (▶ Fig. 3.6).

Pulmonary infarcts may result from pulmonary arterial occlusion. These appear on CTPA as peripheral nonenhancing wedge-shaped opacities (▶ Fig. 3.7). Supporting features include internal lucency (air) within the wedge-shaped opacity, consistent with cavitation within the infarct, in

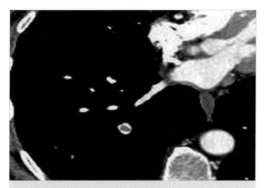

Fig. 3.5 "Polo mint" sign of a partial filling defect.

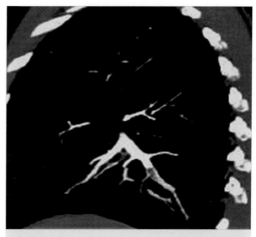

Fig. 3.6 "Tram track" appearance of a filling defect on longitudinal views of the pulmonary arteries.

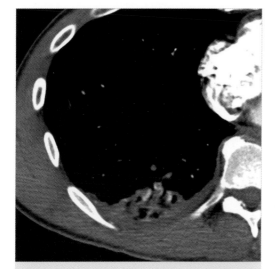

Fig. 3.7 Wedge-shaped opacity with central lucency suggestive of pulmonary infarct.

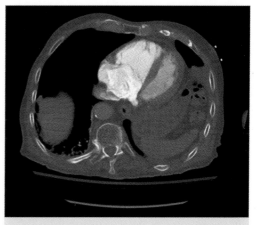

Fig. 3.8 Right ventricular strain pattern. The right ventricle is dilated with respect to the left and the interventricular septum is deviated to the left.

cases of old pulmonary infarcts. In the absence of a filling defect within the pulmonary arterial system, these findings are not specific for pulmonary embolism and may reflect other causes of pulmonary consolidation. In this case, additional evaluation with V/Q scanning or repeat CTPA may be indicated.

Pulmonary embolism can lead to right ventricular (RV) dysfunction and pulmonary arterial hypertension. Recognition of RV dysfunction is vital as it is a predictor of morbidity and mortality. A ratio of RV to left ventricular diameter in short axis greater than 1, deviation of the interventricular septum, increased azygos vein diameter, increased

SVC diameter, and increased pulmonary artery diameter are all signs of RV dysfunction (▶ Fig. 3.8). Clot burden does not appear to be predictive of patients' mortality.[27,28]

3.2.4 Pitfalls

Misdiagnosis of pulmonary embolism or missed pulmonary embolism can result from a multitude of technical and interpretive errors. The most common technical error is respiratory motion during image acquisition, accounting for 42% of misdiagnosed PE[29]

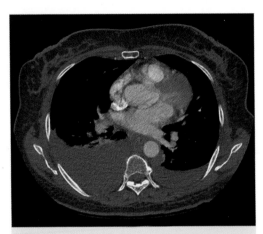

Fig. 3.9 Motion artifact in the left lower lobe causes an artifactual filling defect.

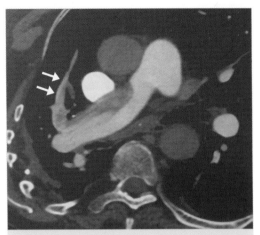

Fig. 3.10 Deep inspiration before contrast injection leads to differential opacification of pulmonary arteries. (arrows depict pseudofilling defect in the pulmonary artery, due to influx of unopacified blood).

(▶ Fig. 3.9). Cardiac motion can also result in erroneous filling defects. Streak artifact results from tubes, lines, or even the patient, if the patient's arms are at their side. Consequently, it is imperative that all extraneous metals be removed from the patient when possible and that the arms be placed above the patient's head. Deep inspiration prior to scanning results in decreased intrathoracic pressure, which draws unopacified blood into the right heart. This can result in mixing of contrast, which may appear as filling defect (▶ Fig. 3.10). This can be prevented by instructing the patient to take a shallow inspiration prior to scanning. Failure to trigger image acquisition at the appropriate time can result in reduced opacification of pulmonary arteries. This can lead to apparent filling defects, particularly in segmental and subsegmental vessels.

3.2.5 Special Considerations

Iodinated contrast agents pose their own potential risks, most importantly allergic reactions and contrast-induced nephropathy (CIN). In patients with a history of allergic reaction to iodinated contrast agents, it is imperative to determine the severity of their reaction. In the case of mild and moderate reactions, the patient can be premedicated with steroids prior to contrast administration. The American College of Radiology contrast manual provides specific guidelines on nonemergent and emergent premedication that include 50 mg of oral prednisone at 13, 7, and 1 hour prior to contrast administration or IV corticosteroid administration

4 to 5 hours prior to contrast administration[30] with a dose of 50-mg diphenhydramine 1 hour prior to contrast administration. Of note, administration of steroids < 2 hours prior to contrast administration has not been shown to be efficacious.

Postcontrast acute kidney injury (PC-AKI) and CIN: PC-AKI refers to any acute kidney injury that occurs in conjunction with IV iodinated contrast administration and includes CIN. CIN is a type of acute tubular necrosis (ATN) defined by an increase in serum creatinine by > 0.3 mg/dL or by 50%, or urine output ≤ 0.5 mg/kg/h for at least 6 hours within 48 hours following contrast administration. While the precise mechanism of CIN is not known, research indicates that it may be related to vasoconstriction and direct toxicity to the tubules. The predominant risk factor for CIN is underlying severe renal insufficiency. There are multiple strategies to reduce the risk of CIN. Volume expansion using 0.9% saline is the main strategy in high-risk patients and is the only strategy that is currently supported by literature. N-acetylcysteine (NAc) has not been shown to reduce the risk of CIN and is not routinely administered prior to contrast administration. Finally, use of iso-osmolar contrast agents such as iodixanol has not been shown to decrease CIN versus low osmolar contrast media (LOCM).[30]

Pregnancy is associated with an increase in the risk of venous thrombosis, which is related to venous stasis and a hypercoagulable state associated with pregnancy. Clinical diagnosis of pulmonary embolism in pregnant patients is hindered by physiologic changes of pregnancy, including tachycardia, tachypnea, and lower extremity edema. Consequently, clinical decision tools are difficult to apply. D-dimer becomes elevated, which can lead to false-positive results. The American Thoracic Society has developed guidelines for imaging of pregnant patients based on symptoms and clinical suspicion.[31] CTPA is indicated if a patient has an abnormal chest radiograph or if a V/Q scan is nondiagnostic. Fetal doses of less than 50 mGy are thought to be inconsequential, although no safe fetal radiation dose has been established. Fetal radiation exposures in CTPA and V/Q scanning are similar. However, maternal exposure is greater in CTPA than in V/Q scan. Fetal radiation exposure during CTPA occurs via direct and scattered radiation. Dose reduction and shielding techniques should be implemented to reduce the effective dose to the mother and the fetus. A reduced-dose protocol includes decreasing the scanning range to include from the aortic arch to the diaphragm and reducing kVp and mA to 100.[32] Ingestion of oral barium attenuates the radiation dose to the fetus.[33] Lead shielding has also been shown to reduce fetal radiation dose.[34]

Radiation exposure is a consideration for every patient undergoing CTPA. The average dose of CTPA using a standard protocol is about 5 mSv. Maximum tube voltage can be reduced to 100 kVp without loss of diagnostic accuracy, which decreases the effective dose by 44%.[32]

CT venography (CTV) of the pelvis can be performed to diagnose DVT of the pelvic veins. However, diagnostic yield of adding either CTV or ultrasound for diagnosis of VTE is relatively low.[35] Therefore, CTV of the pelvis should be performed only in selected cases, as it carries significant radiation exposure. Patients who benefit the most from this study include those in the ICU, whose CTPA quality is more likely to be suboptimal. Patients who have undergone recent pelvic surgery may also benefit, as it provides direct visualization of the deep pelvic vessels. Finally, patients with lower extremity casts cannot undergo sonographic evaluation and therefore may require CTV when they present with the appropriate pretest probability.

3.3 Nuclear Medicine

Current utilization of V/Q scans is limited to patients with renal disease, contrast allergies, or morbidly obese patients,[19,36] as CTPA has been shown to be an accurate and robust technique in PE evaluation.

Although this section is dedicated to V/Q scanning, newer methods of utilizing radiopharmaceuticals have been developed and/or retooled for evaluating DVT. Radiolabeled peptides were developed in recent years, specifically for the detection of DVT with ^{99m}Tc–apcitide gaining the most notoriety demonstrating high sensitivity and specificity in acute DVT; however, it failed to prove PE in 83% of patients with known embolus.[37] Similarly, FDG positron emission tomography (PET)/CT has gained recent success for detection of DVT, although further evaluation of this technique is needed.[38]

3.3.1 Accuracy of Nuclear Medicine Studies for VTE Diagnosis

High-probability V/Q scan can detect the presence of PE with a sensitivity of 77.4% and a specificity of 97.7%.[19] Adding single-photon emission computed tomography (SPECT) increases test sensitivity by improving upon segmental defect detection by 13% and subsegmental defect detection by 80%.[39]

3.3.2 Indication

Similar to CTPA, the patient's pretest probability of PE is calculated by the clinical team using decision-making tools including Wells' criteria, Geneva criteria, and PERC score.[20,21,22] A review by Metter et al summarized nuclear medicine evaluation of PE, including indications for V/Q scanning.[40] If there is a high clinical and biochemical concerns for PE (using decision-making tools and D-dimer), a chest radiograph should be obtained first. If the chest radiograph is normal or near normal, a V/Q scan is indicated with CTPA as a reasonable alternative. In patients in whom CTPA is contraindicated due to renal insufficiency, contrast allergy or morbid obesity V/Q scan can be performed instead. In patients with significantly abnormal chest radiographs or those who are clinically unstable, CTPA is the preferred alternative.

3.3.3 Technique

Evaluation of PE with V/Q scan is a multistep process. A chest X-ray should be obtained prior to the V/Q scan to evaluate the anatomy and allow for comparison of findings per PIOPED II and Prospective Investigative Study of Acute Pulmonary Embolism

Diagnosis (PISAPED) recommendations. For the ventilation scan, the radiopharmaceutical most often used is [99mTc]–diethylenetriamine pentaacetic acid (DTPA),[39] although [133Xe] is used in some academic centers because of its ability to assess all phases of ventilation and ability to provide physiological information, particularly in obstructive airway disease.[39,41] The aerosol is delivered through a nebulizer and mouthpiece with the nose occluded as the patient is breathing and multiple images are taken, in the supine position for [99mTc] and upright for [133Xe]. A minimum of six planar images are captured with the gamma camera of both lungs from the posterior, anterior, left posterior oblique (LPO), right posterior oblique (RPO), left anterior oblique (LAO), and right anterior oblique (RAO) positions for comparison to perfusion imaging taken from the same positions.

The perfusion scan utilizes [99mTc]-macroaggregated albumin (MAA). If [99mTc] DTPA is used, the ventilation scan is performed first with a dose that is considerably lower than the [99mTc]-MAA to ensure that an adequate perfusion phase scan is performed. [133Xe] ventilation scan is frequently performed first; however, at some institutions, the perfusion is performed first allowing for the scenario of a normal perfusion scan with a normal chest X-ray, which then could predicate the omission of the ventilation scan.[39] Disadvantages of the "perfusion-first" method are that if the perfusion scan is nondiagnostic the background activity would contribute to the subsequent ventilation scan, further complicating the study. For the perfusion scan, the patient is placed in the supine position during normal respiration. The [99mTc]-MAA dose is injected intravenously and images are taken in six planes as discussed previously.

The addition of SPECT imaging has emerged over recent years to aid in the detection of pulmonary embolus. Limited to [99mTc] DTPA, this allows the overlapping lung parenchyma to be better assessed in comparison to planar imaging, especially at the subsegmental levels using a gamma camera that captures multiple 2D images over multiple planes and processes them into a 3D rendering. To build upon the V/Q SPECT, low-dose CT has been introduced, allowing for mapping of the perfusion defect to CT imaging and increasing specificity further.

3.3.4 Imaging Features

Study results are reported in terms of pulmonary embolism probability. Ventilation and perfusion imaging are obtained with a preceding chest radiograph although through the PIOPED findings by Sostman et al, ventilation scans are superfluous in most patients when evaluating for PE with a normal chest radiograph.[41] The result of this is that both ventilation and perfusion scans are obtained with the ventilation portion utilized for equivocal cases where body habitus or chronic lung disease may provide information on the ventilation portion.

In a study with high probability of PE, or "PE present," two or more segments of perfusion scan–chest radiograph mismatch (two or more perfusion defects) can be identified (▶ Fig. 3.11). In a study with very low probability of PE, or "PE absent," there can be up to three small perfusion defects or one perfusion defect smaller than a matched radiographic lesion, as well as a single mid- or upper zone segment perfusion scan–chest radiograph mismatch (▶ Fig. 3.12). Multiple radiographic findings not overtly apparent on the accompanying perfusion scan can equal low probability as well including prominent hilum, cardiomegaly, elevated hemidiaphragm, linear atelectasis, and pleural effusions, in at least one-third of a pleural cavity.[41] In all other instances, the study is termed "nondiagnostic" or "intermediate probability."

3.3.5 Pitfalls

During perfusion imaging, blood clotting can occur in the syringe during [99mTc]-MAA injection causing

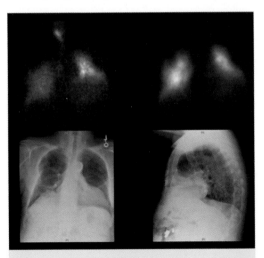

Fig. 3.11 An 86-year-old man with a history of chronic lung disease (CLD) matched small segmental defects in the lung apices corresponding to a large apical bullous seen on the chest radiograph = low likelihood ratio for recent pulmonary emboli.

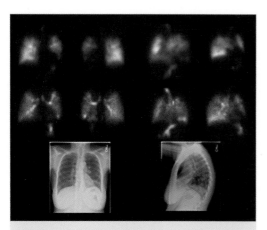

Fig. 3.12 A 54-year-old woman with sarcoidosis with normal chest X-ray and LLL-matched perfusion defects concerning with high probability pulmonary emboli (PE) in left lower lobe.

hotspots on perfusion imaging. Abnormal comparability can be seen between ventilation and perfusion scans secondary to positioning differences and changes in the respiration cycle, given the scans are obtained at two separate time points. Uptake in the thyroid and kidneys may be visualized in cases of right to left shunts.[39] Finally, because the high sensitivity and specificity of the modified PIOPED II criteria rely upon a lack of significant chest X-ray findings, lung pathology such as pneumonia, atelectasis, or even diffuse lung disease may obscure results of the V/Q scan and render a study nondiagnostic.

3.3.6 Special Considerations

Chronic cardiopulmonary concerns can prove problematic in the V/Q scan interpretation. Some of them can be mitigated. For example, in the case of patients with acute obstructive lung disease (chronic obstructive pulmonary disease [COPD] exacerbation), bronchodilator therapy may improve the accuracy of the V/Q scan via improvements in ventilation. Similarly, patients with acute heart failure exacerbation should be medically optimized prior to V/Q scanning to mitigate nondiagnostic imaging resulting from sequelae of heart failure (pulmonary edema, pleural effusions, etc.).[39]

V/Q SPECT shown to improve detection of pulmonary emboli over planar imaging.[43] in sensitivity,

and, with the addition of CT, increased specificity in initial studies.[43] Despite this, no large prospective study has been performed to assess this methodology compared to planar imaging to establish a standard in the same manner as PIOPED II and PISAPED[44]; thus, the use of SPECT varies by institution.

3.4 Conventional Pulmonary Angiography

Conventional angiographic techniques were initially developed in the early 1960s using IV contrast as opposed to selective catheterization due to concern for dislodging emboli. Selective angiography was later shown to be safe and effective and able to detect peripheral emboli. The advent of digital subtraction angiography led to improved procedure time and reduced volume of contrast. For many years, angiography was the gold standard for the diagnosis of pulmonary embolism. With the advent of multidetector CTPA, which is noninvasive with high sensitivity and specificity, conventional angiography has fallen out of favor as a diagnostic technique. It is now reserved for interventions such as catheter-directed thrombectomy and thrombolysis.

3.4.1 Indication

Given the sensitivity and specificity of CTPA without the need for an invasive procedure, the indications for conventional pulmonary angiography are primarily to facilitate intervention. These indications are described in that dedicated section. Diagnostic pulmonary angiography is still used in preoperative planning in the case of chronic pulmonary embolism. It is also used during planning for intervention of pulmonary arteriovenous malformations and fistulas.

3.4.2 Technique

Pulmonary angiography is performed in a similar fashion to many minimally invasive central venous procedures. Briefly, central venous access is obtained through either the internal jugular or common femoral veins. A 6- to 7-Fr sheath can be used, depending on catheter selection. Pressures should be measured in the right atrium, right ventricle, main pulmonary artery, and pulmonary capillary wedge pressure. After accessing the pulmonary

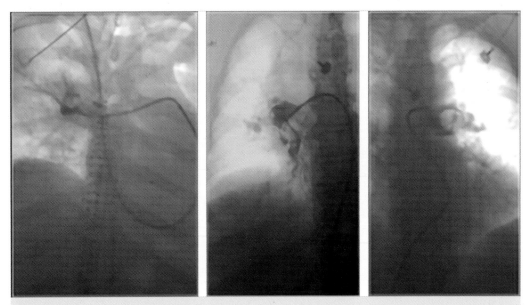

Fig. 3.13 Central main right pulmonary artery and segmental clot demonstrating pulmonary emboli.

artery, angiographic images may be obtained. Injection rates vary based on the vessel being interrogated. A rate of 25 to 30 mL/s for 2 seconds should be used for the main pulmonary artery, 15 to 20 mL/s for 2 seconds for the left and right pulmonary arteries, and 5 to 10 mL/s for 2 seconds for lobar and segmental branches. Extreme care should be taken in performing large-volume power injections in patients with acutely elevated pulmonary pressures, as the increased afterload of the contrast can precipitate acute cardiovascular collapse. Anteroposterior images of each lung and oblique images of the lower lobes should be obtained, with additional images taken at the radiologist's discretion. The frame rate for acquisition of images can also be increased, particularly in patients who are unable to suspend their respiration while imaging.

3.4.3 Imaging Features

As described by Dalen et al in 1971, angiographic abnormalities in pulmonary embolism include intraluminal filling defects, cutoffs of arteries, areas of oligemia, and asymmetric contrast flow[45] (▶ Fig. 3.13).

3.4.4 Pitfalls

Accuracy of pulmonary angiogram is shown to be high in proximal pulmonary artery branches but diminishes in higher-order pulmonary artery branches where branches overlap and can make visualization of filling defects difficult to assess.[46] As in CTPA, respiratory motion can also reduce the sensitivity of this technique.

3.4.5 Special Consideration

Given the rise of CTPA and V/Q scans for PE and ultrasound for DVT, angiography is rarely performed for diagnosis and generally reserved for the cases which intervention will be performed (i.e., thrombectomy or thrombolysis).

References

[1] Heng Tan C, Bedi D, Vikram R. Sonography of thrombosis of the deep veins of the extremities: clinical perspectives and imaging review. J Clin Ultrasound. 2012; 40(1):31–43

[2] Raghavendra BN, Rosen RJ, Lam S, Riles T, Horii SC. Deep venous thrombosis: detection by high-resolution real-time ultrasonography. Radiology. 1984; 152(3):789–793

[3] Talbot S. Use of real-time imaging in identifying deep venous obstruction: a preliminary report. Bruit. 1982; 6:41–42

[4] Beyer J, Schellong S. Deep vein thrombosis: current diagnostic strategy. Eur J Intern Med. 2005; 16(4):238–246

[5] Segal JB, Eng J, Tamariz LJ, Bass EB. Review of the evidence on diagnosis of deep venous thrombosis and pulmonary embolism. Ann Fam Med. 2007; 5(1):63–73

[6] Gottlieb RH, Widjaja J, Tian L, Rubens DJ, Voci SL. Calf sonography for detecting deep venous thrombosis in symptomatic patients: experience and review of the literature. J Clin Ultrasound. 1999; 27(8):415–420

[7] Cogo A, Lensing AW, Wells P, Prandoni P, Büller HR. Noninvasive objective tests for the diagnosis of clinically suspected deep-vein thrombosis. Haemostasis. 1995; 25(1–2):27–39

[8] Wells PS, Lensing AW, Davidson BL, Prins MH, Hirsh J. Accuracy of ultrasound for the diagnosis of deep venous thrombosis in asymptomatic patients after orthopedic surgery. A meta-analysis. Ann Intern Med. 1995; 122(1):47–53

[9] Kearon C, Julian JA, Newman TE, Ginsberg JS. Noninvasive diagnosis of deep venous thrombosis. McMaster Diagnostic Imaging Practice Guidelines Initiative. Ann Intern Med. 1998; 128(8):663–677

[10] Di Nisio M, Van Sluis GL, Bossuyt PMM, Büller HR, Porreca E, Rutjes AW. Accuracy of diagnostic tests for clinically suspected upper extremity deep vein thrombosis: a systematic review. J Thromb Haemost. 2010; 8(4):684–692

[11] Fowkes FJ, Price JF, Fowkes FG. Incidence of diagnosed deep vein thrombosis in the general population: systematic review. Eur J Vasc Endovasc Surg. 2003; 25(1):1–5

[12] White RH. The epidemiology of venous thromboembolism. Circulation. 2003; 107(23) Suppl 1:I4–I8

[13] Wells PS. Integrated strategies for the diagnosis of venous thromboembolism. J Thromb Haemost. 2007; 5 Suppl 1: 41–50

[14] Le Gal G, Carrier M, Rodger M. Clinical decision rules in venous thromboembolism. Best Pract Res Clin Haematol. 2012; 25(3):303–317

[15] Guideline developed in collaboration with the American College of Radiology, Society of Pediatric Radiology, Society of Radiologists in Ultrasound. AIUM practice guideline for the performance of peripheral venous ultrasound examinations. J Ultrasound Med. 2015; 34(8):1–9

[16] Hamper UM, DeJong MR, Scoutt LM. Ultrasound evaluation of the lower extremity veins. Radiol Clin North Am. 2007; 45 (3):525–547, ix

[17] Hanley M, Donahue J, Rybicki FJ, et al. ACR Appropriateness Criteria: Suspected Lower Extremity Deep Venous Thrombosis [online publication]. Reston, VA: American College of Radiology; 2013

[18] Remy-Jardin M, Remy J, Wattinne L, Giraud F. Central pulmonary thromboembolism: diagnosis with spiral volumetric CT with the single-breath-hold technique: comparison with pulmonary angiography. Radiology. 1992; 185(2):381–387

[19] Sostman HD, Stein PD, Gottschalk A, Matta F, Hull R, Goodman L. Acute pulmonary embolism: sensitivity and specificity of ventilation-perfusion scintigraphy in PIOPED II study. Radiology. 2008; 246(3):941–946

[20] Kline JA, Mitchell AM, Kabrhel C, Richman PB, Courtney DM. Clinical criteria to prevent unnecessary diagnostic testing in emergency department patients with suspected pulmonary embolism. J Thromb Haemost. 2004; 2(8):1247–1255

[21] Le Gal G, Righini M, Roy PM, et al. Prediction of pulmonary embolism in the emergency department: the revised Geneva score. Ann Intern Med. 2006; 144(3):165–171

[22] Wells PS, Anderson DR, Rodger M, et al. Excluding pulmonary embolism at the bedside without diagnostic imaging: management of patients with suspected pulmonary embolism presenting to the emergency department by using a simple clinical model and d-dimer. Ann Intern Med. 2001; 135(2): 98–107

[23] Wells PS, Anderson DR, Rodger M, et al. Evaluation of D-dimer in the diagnosis of suspected deep-vein thrombosis. N Engl J Med. 2003; 349(13):1227–1235

[24] Bettmann MA, Baginski SG, White RD, et al. ACR Appropriateness Criteria® acute chest pain: suspected pulmonary embolism. J Thorac Imaging. 2012; 27(2):W28–W31

[25] Stein PD, Woodard PK, Weg JG, et al. PIOPED II Investigators. Diagnostic pathways in acute pulmonary embolism: recommendations of the PIOPED II Investigators. Radiology. 2007; 242(1):15–21

[26] Wittram C, Maher MM, Yoo AJ, Kalra MK, Shepard JA, McLoud TC. CT angiography of pulmonary embolism: diagnostic criteria and causes of misdiagnosis. Radiographics. 2004; 24(5): 1219–1238

[27] van der Meer RW, Pattynama PMT, van Strijen MJ, et al. Right ventricular dysfunction and pulmonary obstruction index at helical CT: prediction of clinical outcome during 3-month follow-up in patients with acute pulmonary embolism. Radiology. 2005; 235(3):798–803

[28] Ghaye B, Ghuysen A, Willems V, et al. Severe pulmonary embolism:pulmonary artery clot load scores and cardiovascular parameters as predictors of mortality. Radiology. 2006; 239 (3):884–891

[29] Hutchinson BD, Navin P, Marom EM, Truong MT, Bruzzi JF. Overdiagnosis of pulmonary embolism by pulmonary CT angiography. AJR Am J Roentgenol. 2015; 205(2):271–277

[30] ACR Committee on Drugs and Contrast Media. ACR Manual on Contrast Media. Version 10.3. Reston, VA: American College of Radiology; 2017

[31] Leung AN, Bull TM, Jaeschke R, et al. ATS/STR Committee on Pulmonary Embolism in Pregnancy. An official American Thoracic Society/Society of Thoracic Radiology clinical practice guideline: evaluation of suspected pulmonary embolism in pregnancy. Am J Respir Crit Care Med. 2011; 184(10): 1200–1208

[32] Heyer CM, Mohr PS, Lemburg SP, Peters SA, Nicolas V. Image quality and radiation exposure at pulmonary CT angiography with 100- or 120-kVp protocol: prospective randomized study. Radiology. 2007; 245(2):577–583

[33] Yousefzadeh DK, Ward MB, Reft C. Internal barium shielding to minimize fetal irradiation in spiral chest CT: a phantom simulation experiment. Radiology. 2006; 239(3):751–758

[34] Chatterson LC, Leswick DA, Fladeland DA, Hunt MM, Webster ST. Lead versus bismuth-antimony shield for fetal dose reduction at different gestational ages at CT pulmonary angiography. Radiology. 2011; 260(2):560–567

[35] Goodman LR, Sostman HD, Stein PD, Woodard PK. CT venography: a necessary adjunct to CT pulmonary angiography or a waste of time, money, and radiation? Radiology. 2009; 250 (2):327–330

[36] Yazdani M, Lau CT, Lempel JK, et al. Historical evolution of imaging techniques for the evaluation of pulmonary embolism. Radiographics. 2015; 35(4):1245–1262

[37] Dunzinger A, Hafner F, Schaffler G, Piswanger-Soelkner JC, Brodmann M, Lipp RW. 99mTc-apcitide scintigraphy in patients with clinically suspected deep venous thrombosis and

pulmonary embolism. Eur J Nucl Med Mol Imaging. 2008; 35 (11):2082–2087

[38] Hess S, Madsen PH, Iversen ED, Frifelt JJ, Høilund-Carlsen PF, Alavi A. Efficacy of FDG PET/CT imaging for venous thromboembolic disorders: preliminary results from a prospective, observational pilot study. Clin Nucl Med. 2015; 40(1):e23–e26

[39] Parker JA, Coleman RE, Grady E, et al. Society of Nuclear Medicine. SNM practice guideline for lung scintigraphy 4.0. J Nucl Med Technol. 2012; 40(1):57–65

[40] Metter D, Tulchinsky M, Freeman LM. Current status of ventilation-perfusion scintigraphy for suspected pulmonary embolism. AJR Am J Roentgenol. 2017; 208(3):489–494

[41] Mettler FA, Guiberteau MJ. Respiratory system. In: Essentials of Nuclear Medicine Imaging. 6th ed. Philadelphia, PA: Elsevier/Saunders; 2012:197–219

[42] Stein PD, Sostman HD, Matta F. Critical review of SPECT imaging in pulmonary embolism. Clin Transl Imaging. 2014; 2: 379–390

[43] Reinartz P, Wildberger JE, Schaefer W, Nowak B, Mahnken AH, Buell U. Tomographic imaging in the diagnosis of pulmonary embolism: a comparison between V/Q lung scintigraphy in SPECT technique and multislice spiral CT. J Nucl Med. 2004; 45 (9):1501–1508

[44] Sostman HD, Miniati M, Gottschalk A, Matta F, Stein PD, Pistolesi M. Sensitivity and specificity of perfusion scintigraphy combined with chest radiography for acute pulmonary embolism in PIOPED II. J Nucl Med. 2008; 49(11): 1741–1748

[45] Dalen JE, Brooks HL, Johnson LW, Meister SG, Szucs MM, Jr, Dexter L. Pulmonary angiography in acute pulmonary embolism: indications, techniques, and results in 367 patients. Am Heart J. 1971; 81(2):175–185

[46] Stein PD, Athanasoulis C, Alavi A, et al. Complications and validity of pulmonary angiography in acute pulmonary embolism. Circulation. 1992; 85(2):462–468

Chapter 4

Catheter-Directed Thrombolysis Treatment of Deep Venous Thrombosis

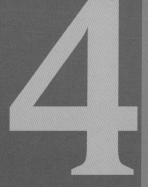

4 Catheter-Directed Thrombolysis Treatment of Deep Venous Thrombosis

Dana Safavian and John Fritz Angle

Keywords: lysis, mechanical thrombectomy

The annual rate of venous thromboembolic events (VTEs) over the period 1985 to 2009 was estimated at 142 per 100,000 persons, with an associated annual healthcare cost of over $10 billion in the United States. Of the VTEs, 50% presented as lower extremity deep venous thrombosis (DVT) alone, 30% as pulmonary embolism (PE) alone, and 20% as DVT and PE.[1] Even with aggressive multispecialty treatment of PE, 30-day mortality is nearly 5 to 20% in high-risk patients.[2]

Long-term complications are quite common in patients with VTE. For patients suffering from PE, recurrence was an important cause of mortality in a Danish study that followed up patients who suffered from a PE episode for 3 years.[3] The general lifetime recurrence rate of DVTs is about 25%.[1] Patients who suffer from unprovoked DVT have a substantially higher 10-year risk of recurrence: above 50% if not treated with extended duration anticoagulation. Patients who suffer DVT in the setting of modifiable risk factors have a 10-year recurrence rate of 20%.[4]

Post-thrombotic syndrome (PTS) is the most debilitating long-term sequalae of DVT. It manifests as chronic valvular dysfunction leading to limb pain, swelling, heaviness, and fatigue.[5] In some cases, it progresses to stasis dermatitis and limb ulceration. Between 40 and 50% of adult patients develop PTS over 2 years after the onset of their DVT symptoms.[6] The risk of PTS is approximately 25% in children and adolescents with DVT.[7]

The exact pathophysiology of PTS is unknown. Venous hypertension is thought to play a pivotal role in this process.[8] The increased intraluminal pressure is thought to reduce tissue perfusion, leading to increased vascular permeability and edema.[9] Two pathological mechanisms contribute to venous hypertension: acute and chronic venous obstruction and valvular dysfunction.[10] Inflammation may also be responsible in the development of PTS by delaying thrombus resolution and by inducing wall fibrosis, both of which further promotes valvular reflux.[11,12] Genetic factors controlling vascular wall remodeling can also contribute to vascular injury and PTS.[13]

4.1 Anatomy

Lower extremity DVT events are classified based on their anatomic locations as proximal DVT (involving the popliteal, femoral, and iliac veins) or distal DVT (involving the calf veins including the peroneal, posterior and anterior tibial, and muscular veins) (▶ Fig. 4.1).[14] In a study of 885 patients with venographic evidence of DVTs, Ouriel et al found peroneal vein was the most common site of thrombosis. Postoperative DVTs were shown to be more frequently associated with distal clots. DVTs developing in the setting of malignancy, however, were more frequently proximal and often right sided. Proximal, left-sided DVTs were common in patients with no identifiable DVT risk factors, presumably as a result of undiagnosed left iliac vein webs.[15] Liu et al demonstrated in orthopedic patients that the incidence of left proximal DVT is higher and more symptomatic if there is iliac vein compression.[16]

Proximal DVTs carry a higher risk of developing into PE and are therefore a greater concern. The primary venous outflow of the legs is dependent on the patency of iliofemoral veins. The presence of thrombus burden in iliofemoral veins is detected in 25% of symptomatic DVT patients.[6] The presence of thrombus in one or both of these veins is called iliofemoral deep vein thrombosis (IFDVT). IFDVT occludes the collateral venous outflow of the legs leading to venous congestion and severe clinical symptoms of DVT in the leg.[17] The IFDVT subgroup is associated with worse prognosis than the larger group of proximal DVT. It has been shown that patients with symptomatic IFDVT have a twofold increase in PTS over a 2-year follow-up period and a 2.4-fold increase in the risk of recurrent venous thromboembolism over a 3-month follow-up period compared to those with distal DVT.[6,18]

Isolated distal deep vein thrombosis (IDDVT) refers to another type of lower extremity DVT which generally carries a better prognosis than IFDVT.[19] IDDVT is defined as thrombosis of one or more of the deep calf veins without reaching the popliteal vein. The deep calf veins (also known as below knee veins or deep distal veins) include the paired peroneal, posterior tibial, and anterior tibial veins, which run along the homonymous arteries, as well

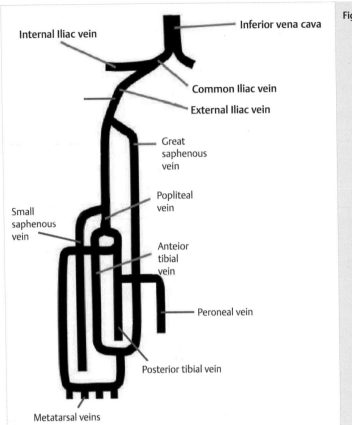

Fig. 4.1 Venous network of the leg.

Internal Iliac vein

Inferior vena cava

Common Iliac vein

External Iliac vein

Great saphenous vein

Popliteal vein

Small saphenous vein

Anteior tibial vein

Peroneal vein

Posterior tibial vein

Metatarsal veins

as two groups of muscle veins, the soleal and gastrocnemius muscle veins. Soleal muscle veins drain into the posterior tibial vein and the gastrocnemius muscle veins connect to the peroneal veins. Although there is large degree of variability in the anatomy of these veins, they usually merge in a trifurcation area before forming the popliteal vein.

4.2 Diagnosis

In the clinical setting, the initial diagnosis of DVT is almost exclusively made by ultrasonographic investigation of the veins, using lack of vein compressibility as the primary marker for thrombosis. Compression ultrasonography (CUS) examination protocols to diagnose DVTs may be serial (proximal) or complete CUS (proximal and distal). The proximal CUS method involves examining only the veins proximal to the trifurcation. The subject is first examined in the supine position from the groin to the Hunter's canal to assess the common, deep, and superficial femoral veins. The patient is then placed in the prone position and the popliteal

vein is examined to the trifurcation. This approach is based on the assumption that distal DVTs pose a smaller risk of complications compared to proximal lesions. To eliminate the risk of potential distal DVT growth with late involvement of proximal vessels, the CUS investigation should be repeated during 1- to 2-week time period following the initial investigation in high-risk patients (those with high clinical probability and/or positive D-dimer assay) to detect and treat proximal thrombi.

In the complete CUS examination, all deep veins of the symptomatic leg are examined in a single study. The complete CUS involves investigating the proximal veins as mentioned above followed by investigating the calf veins with the patient in the sitting position. Complete CUS has a larger degree of inter-observer variability than proximal vein CUS. It also requires specifically trained operators and is more time consuming and costly. Furthermore, there have been studies that questioned the accuracy of the complete CUS strategy.[20,21] Both examination protocols have been shown to be effective and safe, and they are widely used in the clinical setting.[22]

4.3 Anticoagulation

According to the American College of Chest Physicians guidelines on antithrombotic treatments published in 2008 both proximal and distal DVTs should be treated with immediate anticoagulant for at least 3 months.[23] However, the 2012 edition of the guidelines states patients with acute isolated distal DVT of the leg, without severe symptoms or risk factors for extension, should be followed by serial imaging of the deep veins over the period of 2 weeks following presentation without initial anticoagulation (Grade 2C).[24] The risk factors considered in the guidelines include presence of positive D-dimer, a thrombosis that is close to the proximal veins, thrombus length > 5 cm, multiple vein involvement, maximum vein diameter of > 7 mm, lack of reversible provoking factor for DVT, active cancer, history of VTE, and inpatient status. Patients with symptomatic IDDVT or risk factors for extension should undergo initial anticoagulation (Grade 2C).[25]

The 2012 version of National Clinical Guideline Centre recommendations did not mention treatment for IDDVT since the guidelines are focused on proximal DVT rather than deep calf vein DVT as the latter poses a smaller risk of PTS and embolization to the lungs.[25] In contrast, the International Consensus Statement on Prevention and Treatment of Venous Thromboembolism states that all patients with symptomatic DVT should undergo oral anticoagulation.[26] These differences highlight the broad variabilities in treatment strategies for DVTs and the lower risk associated with direct oral antioagulant (DOAC). The recommended initial anticoagulation dosages for patients presenting with proximal DVT are as follows:

- Intravenous (IV) unfractionated heparin bolus of 80 units/kg followed by a continuous infusion of 18 units/kg/hour to a target anti-Xa activity (plasma heparin levels of 0.3–0.7 IU/mL for 5–7 days for patients with high-risk IFDVT).[27] Fixed-dose, weight-adjusted subcutaneous unfractionated heparin has also been used in this clinical setting although a limited number of studies have been conducted to support this regimen.[28]
- Subcutaneous low molecular weight heparin with enoxaparin 1 mg/kg twice daily, dalteparin once daily at 200 IU/kg, or tinzaparin once daily at 175 anti-Xa IU/kg.[29]
- Subcutaneous fondaparinux 5 mg daily for patients below 50 kg, 7.5 mg daily for patients weighing 50 to 100 kg, or 10 mg daily for patients weighing > 100 kg.[30,31]

Direct thrombin inhibitors such as IV argatroban or lepirudin must be used in patients with type II heparin-induced thrombocytopenia (HIT). A prospective cohort study showed the safety and efficacy of argatroban in DVT patients without type II HIT as well.[32]

Long-term anticoagulation therapy is used (3 to 6 months for patients with a single episode of DVT, up to a year or even longer for patients with recurrent DVTs, phlegmasia cerulea dolens, or persisting but reversible DVT risk factors) beyond the initial treatment for acute DVT. Previously, vitamin K antagonists (i.e., warfarin with a target international normalized ratio [INR] of 2–3) or low molecular weight heparins (LMWHs) were the only available options for long-term anticoagulation therapy. However, these medications are associated with numerous limitations such as slow onset and offset of action, a narrow therapeutic window, unpredictable pharmacokinetics with significant interactions with food and other medications, and the required regular monitoring.[33,34] Direct oral antioagulants (DOACs) address several of these limitations including more predictable pharmacokinetics with a faster onset of action and shorter half-life, and fewer drug and food interactions and elimination of need for regular monitoring.[35,36]

All four DOACs (rivaroxaban, apixaban, dabigatran, and edoxaban) have been studied for use in long-term anticoagulation in patients with DVT. Rivaroxaban (15 mg twice daily for the first 21 days followed by 20 mg once daily) was noninferior to enoxaparin for treatment of DVT and PE in ODIXa-DVT and EINSTEIN DVT trials.[37,38] RECORD 1–4 trials showed rivaroxaban was more effective in preventing DVTs in arthroplasty patients compared to enoxaparin.[39,40] Apixaban is also noninferior to enoxaparin followed by warfarin in the phase III trial AMPLIFY.[41] HOKUSAI trial showed noninferiority and fewer bleeding complications for edoxaban compared to standard therapy for VTE patients.[42] Dabigatran was found to be noninferior to warfarin in several trials including RE-COVER, RE-MEDY, and RE-NOVATE.[43,44,45] Although this was not consistent in all trials, major (0.3% vs. 0%) and clinically relevant bleeding (5.3% vs. 1.8%; hazard ratio 2.92; 95% confidence interval [CI], 1.52–5.60) were significantly higher in the dabigatran group compared to warfarin in the RE-SONATE trial.[44]

Rivaroxaban,[46] apixaban,[47] edoxaban,[42] and dabigatran[48] were more effective than standard of care in total hip and knee arthroplasty with no increase in the incidence of postoperative bleeding compared to standard of treatment. Rivaroxaban has been FDA approved for acute and long-term treatment of DVT and PE, VTE prophylaxis in total hip or knee arthroplasty, and nonvalvular atrial fibrillation. In 2011, apixaban was approved for prophylaxis of VTE after elective orthopedic operations. It was also approved in July 2014 for the treatment and prevention of relapse of PE and DVT.

4.4 Systemic Thrombolytic Therapy for VTE

Intravenous administration of a fibrinolytic drug in order to achieve thrombus resolution in distant vessels is referred to as systemic thrombolysis. The use of systemic thrombolysis in VTE treatment is controversial. So far 16 randomized controlled trials have been conducted to compare the efficacy of systemic thrombolysis versus anticoagulation alone for the treatment of acute PE. In the Pulmonary Embolism Thrombolysis (PEITHO) study, the largest trial of systemic thrombolysis for submassive PE to date, IV infusion of fibrinolytics was shown to prevent hemodynamic decompensation while it increased the risk of intracranial bleeding.[49]

There is paucity of data on the use of thrombolytics for massive PE due to the high rate of prehospital mortality as well as ethical and practical limitations in randomizing those patients. Overall, the current data does not support a clear strategy for when PE patients should receive thrombolysis versus anticoagulation alone. This is in part because the mortality benefit of systemic fibrinolytic administration for submassive PE can be greatly offset by the increased risk of intracranial bleeding. Therefore, clinicians should tailor their decision on the use of systemic thrombolytics based on the clinical status of the patients. Systemic thrombolysis is advisable for select patients with acute PE who are hemodynamically unstable (massive PE) or who have evidence of right ventricle (RV) dysfunction (submassive PE), for whom fibrinolysis is not contraindicated.

Thrombolytic therapy can also be used for acute DVT to reduce thrombus burden, expedite the restoration of venous flow, and reduce venous congestion.[49] Thrombolysis is crucial in certain clinical scenarios such as the following:

- To resolve the clot burden in acute DVT patients with limb-threatening circulatory compromise (i.e., phlegmasia cerulea dolens) or progressive IVC thrombosis which can potentially lead to PE or visceral organ injury.[50]
- To expedite symptomatic relief in patients who despite anticoagulation therapy demonstrate clinical or anatomic expansion of the symptoms.[51]
- To prevent late sequela of DVT such as venous valvular dysfunction and PTS.[52]

Previous randomized clinical trials have assessed the use of systemic thrombolysis to treat acute proximal DVTs. In studies that compared the use of systemic first-generation fibrinolytic, streptokinase, versus anticoagulation alone, better clot resolution (quantified by venographic assessment of affected veins) was achieved with streptokinase infusion. In a 1979 randomized controlled trial, Elliot et al demonstrated patients treated with systemic streptokinase had a lower rate of PTS development for up to 19 months following acute DVTs compared to those treated with anticoagulation alone (35% vs. 92% respectively, $n = 51$).[53] In 1982, Arnesen et al found that systemic thrombolysis reduces residual thrombus burden (assessed venographically) and PTS for up to 6.5 years following acute DVT.[54] Additionally, Goldhaber et al found in a pooled study of six randomized controlled trials that the incidence of major bleeding complications was much higher in patients treated with systemic streptokinase (14% vs. 4%).[55] It was after this study that the use of systemic streptokinase infusions was restricted to certain clinical situations as discussed above.

Tissue plasminogen activator (rtPA) is a newer and more expansive clot buster with a greater affinity for fibrin compared to streptokinase. Systemic infusion of rtPA has been studied for the treatment of DVT and the findings have been consistent with those of previous studies on streptokinase. In 1990, Turpie et al recruited 59 proximal DVT patients in a randomized controlled trial to compare systemic rtPA versus anticoagulation alone. The study demonstrated above 50% thrombus lysis after a 4-hour systemic rtPA infusion (0.5 mg/kg). It also showed a lower rate of PTS in a 2-year follow-up for patients who achieved above 50% thrombus lysis (25% vs. 56%, $p = 0.07$).[56]

In a multicenter randomized study of 64 patients with proximal DVT, Goldhaber et al corroborated the previous finding of superior efficacy of systemic streptokinase over anticoagulation alone in achieving > 50% thrombus lysis. They used an rtPA infusion rate of 0.05 mg/kg/hour for up to 24 hours, at a maximum total dose of 150 mg. This study also demonstrated the probability of achieving > 50% thrombus lysis was higher in nonocclusive than occlusive clots (59% vs. 14% respectively, $p < 0.005$). Additionally, systemic rtPA infusion achieved only modest thrombolysis (29–58%) in the majority of patients in the two studies mentioned above.[57] These findings suggested systemic fibrinolytic administration through the IV route is unable to consistently achieve therapeutic rtPA concentrations throughout the clot. In the two studies combined ($N = 123$), one nonfatal intracranial and two extracranial hemorrhages happened. Two patients had extracranial bleeding. The use of intermittent, local, IV injection of rtPA (injection of thrombolytics into nearby veins in the affected extremity) has also been studied in a randomized control trial of 137 patients. This method did not show any differences in efficacy or safety profiles between adjacent and distant administration of thrombolytics.[58]

4.5 Catheter-Directed Thrombolysis for DVT

With catheter-directed thrombolysis (CDT), the infusion catheter is used to deliver various thrombolytic regimens directly into the thrombus, achieving higher thrombolytic concentrations in the clot than systemic therapy. CDT is an invasive procedure that uses fluoroscopy to place a multi-sidehole infusion catheter inside a thrombus, and then deliver pulse or drip thrombolytic infusion, with or without additional mechanical thrombectomy. Some advocate the use of an ultrasound wire within the infusion catheter to speed up thrombolysis.[59]

In the CDT approach, after the acute thrombus has been dissolved with several hours of infusion, venographic assessment is performed to identify and treat any residual thrombus or other venous obstructive lesion by balloon angioplasty and/or stent placement. CDT facilitates early thrombus reduction which leads to improved long-term benefits. Percutaneous therapy in the acute phase of venous thrombosis has been shown to reduce the incidence of valvular damage, PTS, and recurrent venous thrombosis.[60]

There are three randomized trials assessing the long-term outcomes of CDT with or without mechanical therapy. Some of the limitations of this

technique include the long infusion times required to lyse extensive DVT (typically 12–24 hours or longer) and the extensive healthcare resources used such as angiography suite time and inpatient observation during thrombolysis. Okrent et al published the first report on the use of CDT to treat IFDVT patients in 1991. Their technique involved obtaining access to the thrombus site under fluoroscopy through an internal jugular approach followed by intra-thrombus urokinase delivery over 68 hours. Adjuvant balloon angioplasty was also done to treat residual webbing.[61] In 1992, Molina et al recruited 11 patients with acute or subacute thrombosis causing phlegmasia cerulean dolens. The patients received intra-thrombus urokinase delivery from an internal jugular venous approach which achieved thrombus resolution in 95% of the cases at a median therapeutic duration of 2.9 days (range 2–4 days). They also treated residual stenosis with balloon angioplasty. All patients reported symptomatic improvement, and no major bleeding or PE was reported. Four patients had an inferior vena cava filter (IVCF) placed in conjunction with the procedure.[62] The success of these early reports underscored the importance of pharmacological thrombolysis and treating the underlying venous stenosis. In 1994, Semba and Dake incorporated venous stenting in the treatment of DVT associated stenosis. They used Wallstents (Boston Scientific, Natick, MA, USA) for this purpose.[63]

In 1997, Bjarnason et al established the importance of early intervention in improving rates of the treatment. If treated within 1 week of symptom onset, technical success was 86%. The success rate dropped to 79% for symptoms of 1 to 2 weeks duration, and 33% if symptoms started more than 4 weeks prior to initiation of CDT.[64]

The first multicenter registry evaluating treatment outcomes of CDT was established in 1999 which included 63 centers across the United States. The study involved urokinase CDT treatment of 312 limbs with either acute (≤ 10 days) or chronic thrombosis (> 10 days) proximal DVTs (from the inferior vena cava to the popliteal veins). The overall primary patency rate was 65% at 6 months and 60% at 12 months. The efficacy of femoral–popliteal was lower than iliofemoral CDT with the 1-year patency rates at 47 and 64%, respectively ($P < 0.01$). Patients who received a stent (33%) had a higher patency rate at 1 year (74% vs. 53%, $P < 0.001$).[65]

Mewissen et al established a thrombus burden scoring tool in 1999 to quantify the degree of thrombotic obstruction and the efficacy of thrombolysis. With this tool, venous lesions were initially scored on a scale of 0 to 2 based on patency (0 = open vein, 1 = partially occluded vein, 2 = totally occluded vein). This grading tool has subsequently evolved to better quantify and express the percentage of thrombolysis accomplished (grade I ≤ 50%, grade II = 50–90%, grade III = complete thrombolysis). This scoring system has been very effective for performing inter-study comparisons.[65]

Elsharawy et al performed the first randomized controlled trial to study efficacy and safety of CDT for DVT patients. They demonstrated improved venous patency rates at 6 months (72% vs. 12%, $P < 0.0001$) and lower venous insufficiency rates (41% vs. 11%, $P < 0.04$) in patients who received streptokinase versus anticoagulant alone.[66]

A larger CaVenT trial randomized 189 patients with thrombi involving lower extremity venous system to either combined rtPA CDT and anticoagulation or anticoagulation alone (plus compression stockings). The study demonstrated higher patency rates for CDT and anticoagulation group at 6 months follow-up (64% vs. 36%, absolute risk reduction of 28.2%, 95% CI: 9.7–46.7%, $P = 0.004$). The incidence of major bleeding associated with thrombolytics was reasonably low at 4% and there were no PEs. Although effective in reducing outflow obstruction assessed by venous plethysmography (20% vs. 49%, absolute risk reduction of 29% vs. 95%, CI: 20.0–38.0%, $P = 0.004$), CDT did not reduce the incidence of PTS in 6-month post-treatment follow-up. There was statistically significant reduction in the incidence of PTS in the 5-year follow-up study (43%; 95% CI 33-53 versus 71%; 95% CI 61-79). However, there was not a significant difference in quality of life scores and the incidence of severe PTS was low (5% versus 1%).[67]

The ATTRACT trial is the largest trial with 692 symptomatic first-time proximal DVT of 14 days or fewer days. The incidence of post thrombotic syndrome (PTS), the main outcome, was 47% in the CDT group and 48% in the control group at 2 years ($P = 0.56$). This lack of significant difference was very surprising to venous disease physicians. However, the study did show that moderate-to-severe PTS (Villalta > = 10) occurred in 18% of patients in the CDT group and 24% of those in the control group ($P = 0.04$). In addition, PTS scores were lower in the CDT group than in the control group at follow-up ($P < 0.01$). Thrombolysis led to more major bleeding events within 10 days

(1.7% vs. 0.3%, $P = 0.049$). There was no significant difference in recurrent VTE (12% in the CDT group and 8% in the control group, $P = 0.09$). Like with the CaVenT trial, disease specific quality of life change from baseline to 24 months was not significantly different ($P = 0.08$).

CDT lowers the fibrinolytic dose required to achieve thrombus clearance, thus reducing the risk of major intracranial and extracranial bleeds. This greatly reduces the risk to benefit ratio of this method.[68] An early prospective multicenter registry demonstrated major bleeding complications in 11% of DVT patients treated with urokinase CDT. More recent studies have utilized infusions of rtPA at low doses (0.5–1.0 mg/hour) which led to a lower incidence of major bleeding (only 3–4%). The third major randomized trial is the CAVA trial (Ultrasound-Accelerated Catheter-Directed Thrombolysis Versus Anticoagulation for the Prevention of Post-Thrombotic Syndrome). This was a randomized trial of 184 acute ilio-femoral DVT with primary outcome of PTS (Villalta score ≥ 5 on 2 occasions, ≥ 3 months apart, or venous ulceration) at 1-year. They found PTS in 22 (29%) in the CDT versus 26 (35%) in the control group (OR 0·75; p = 0.42). In addition, major bleeding occurred in four patients (5%) in the intervention group, and none in the control group. Clearly, further work is needed to define the role of CDT. There remains clinical application of CDT in iliac thrombus, thrombus associated with significant acute symptoms, and in those with known hypercoagulable disorders.[69,70,71,72,73]

There has been tremendous progress made in endovascular removal of acute thrombosis of the iliac and femoral veins since the development of CDT method in 1991. in patients with popliteal and calf thrombi, an infusion system is commonly inserted into the popliteal vein or posterior tibial vein at the ankle to improve femoral venous inflow. CDT by itself is a slow and expensive procedure, which takes an average of 3 days during which time the patient requires close monitoring for any signs of bleeding or PE.[70,72]

Currently, the most commonly used fibrinolytic in the clinical setting to treat DVT is rtPA (Genentech, South San Francisco, CA, USA). Limited use of reteplase (Centocor, Malvern, PA, USA) and tenecteplase (Genentech, South San Francisco, CA, USA) in this setting has also been reported.[71,73,74] Each of these drugs is FDA approved for other indications but is used off-label for DVT lysis. Recombinant tissue plasminogen activator is infused through the infusion catheter at a typical low dose of 0.5 to 1.0 mg/hour. During this time, the patient also receives an IV infusion of unfractionated heparin at subtherapeutic levels. Most centers place the patient in an intensive care or stepdown unit for close monitoring. Hematocrit, partial thromboplastin time (PTT), platelet count, and fibrinogen level are obtained every 6 to 12 hours. If active bleeding is suspected or if laboratory parameters depart from the expected ranges (e.g., PTT > 100 sec, fibrinogen < 100 mg/dL), the fibrinolytic infusion is temporarily or permanently halted.

Treatment progress is monitored at 6 to 24 hours intervals. If only partial thrombolysis is achieved, an angioplasty balloon is used to increase the vessel diameter and enhance thrombolytic contact with the clot. Thrombolytic infusion is then continued. Following the completion of thrombolysis, venography is repeated to visualize any remaining stenotic lesions. Venoplasty and stent placement are then performed as needed. Therapeutic anticoagulation is then restarted, and patients are subsequently transitioned to long-term vitamin K antagonist or newer oral anticoagulant therapy.

4.6 Mechanical Thrombectomy

The introduction of mechanical thrombectomy devices has reduced the amount of time and thrombolytic dosage required to achieve grade II thrombolysis. These devices function through physical disruption and aspiration of thrombotic material. Thrombolytic agents can be administered through the mechanical thrombectomy device (also known as pharmacomechanical thrombectomy [PCMT]) or CDT can be performed as an adjunct treatment following mechanical thrombectomy.[75]

In recent years, PCMT methods involving single session treatments have become available. The Angiojet Rheolytic Thrombectomy Catheter (Possis Medical, Minneapolis, MN, USA) uses the "power-pulse" technique to forcefully spray the thrombolytic drug into the thrombus as it is advanced inside the vessel. Angiojet is then used after a 20- to 30-minute incubation period to aspirate the residual thrombus.[76]

There is increasing usage of mechanical devices for single-visit effective thrombectomy. These include larger-bore aspiration catheters with customized suction capabilities, and nitinol mesh baskets that can scope large amounts of thrombus into a popliteal sheath.[77]

The PEARL registry evaluated the safety and efficacy of AngioJet Thrombectomy (Boston Scientific Corporation, Marlborough, MA, USA). In this study 329 patients with lower extremity DVT underwent a combination of CDT and mechanical thrombectomy using the device (rheolytic thrombectomy [RT] without lytic agent in 4% of patients [13 of 329], PCMT in 35% [115 of 329], PCMT combined with further CDT in 52% [172 of 329], and RT combined with CDT in 9% [29 of 329]). The use of this device reduced the average treatment time (median procedure times for RT alone, PCDT, PCDT/CDT, and RT/CDT were 1.4, 2, 22, and 41 hours, respectively; median procedure time for CDT alone was reported to be 72 hours in earlier studies). Major bleeding occurred in 12 patients (3.6%) but none of them was attributed to the AngioJet device. No PE events were reported in the study.[78]

In the Thrombus Obliteration by Rapid Percutaneous Endovenous Intervention in Deep Venous Occlusion (TORPEDO) trial, 183 patients were randomized to PCMT versus anticoagulation alone. AngioJet (Bayer Healthcare, Warrendale, PA, USA), Trellis (Bacchus Vascular, Santa Clara, CA, USA), and manual aspiration were used in this study. Adjunctive CDT was performed for cases with above 30% residual thrombus. The incidence of PTS at 6 months was significantly less in the PCMT group compared to that of anticoagulation alone (3.4% vs. 27.2%, P < 0.001). Those who did develop PTS had less severe symptoms in the PCMT group. Hospital stay was also significantly lowered with PCMT.[79]

Most recently, the results of the Acute Venous Thrombosis: Thrombus Removal with Adjunctive Catheter-Directed Thrombolysis (ATTRACT) trial were presented at the Society of Interventional Radiology annual meeting in Washington D.C. The primary outcome was PTS at 24 months using the Villalta scale. The trial data showed that patients treated with pharmacomechanical catheter-directed thrombolysis (PCDT) had a 46.7% PTS rate compared with 48.2% in the medical management group at 2 years (p = 0.56). However, PCDT reduced early symptoms and PTS severity; iliofemoral DVT had better results with PCDT than femoropopliteal DVT. The trial showed that PCDT resulted in more major hemorrhage events (1.7%) than in the control arm (0.3%; p = 0.049).[80]

Although there are no peer-reviewed multicenter randomized controlled trials on the outcomes of PCMT, a growing body of evidence from smaller studies demonstrated the safety and efficacy of

CDT or PCMT in DVT patients with clinically severe manifestations of DVT including phlegmasia cerulea dolens, acute IVC thrombosis, or rapid thrombus extension despite conventional anticoagulation therapy. CDT and PCMT have also been shown to improve outcomes in extensive thrombotic lesion involving the common femoral and/or iliac vein. If untreated, IFDVT is associated with a much higher risk of recurrent DVT and PTS.[81,82] Therefore, the treatment planning for each patient should be tailored based on the clinical status and the location and extension of the DVT lesion.

Current guidelines recommend taking into consideration symptom duration, the patient's bleeding risk profile, life-expectancy, and expected activity level following the treatment when deciding on the use of invasive versus noninvasive DVT treatment modalities.[81]

4.7 Who Benefits from Pharmacomechanical Therapy

Improved outcomes are expected in patients with recent onset of DVT symptoms (< 10–14 days).[83] Patients with left-sided IFDVT are likely to have an underlying stenosis (May–Thurner syndrome). Therefore, PCMT along with stenting can be very effective for those patients. Patients with symptom duration of 14 to 28 days usually respond favorably to thrombolysis. However, in most cases they require adjunctive iliac vein stenting to restore flow and improve long-term outcomes.[84]

Invasive thrombolytic therapies are contraindicated in patients with short life-expectancy, higher bleeding risk (e.g., recent surgery, trauma, intracranial lesions, or severe thrombocytopenia), and those who are nonambulatory.[81]

The use of invasive thrombolytic therapies is less clear for the following patient groups:
- Patients with chronic femoropopliteal DVT (> 28 days) due to limited long-term efficacy[84]
- Patients with femoral-popliteal or calf DVT due to less severe symptoms and lower risk of long-term DVT recurrence and sequalae[85]
- Asymptomatic patients with incidental DVT findings due to rarity of PTS development in this patient group[85]

4.8 Upper Extremity

Upper extremity DVT comprise only 5% of all VTE events.[86] Common etiologies include central venous stenosis due to long-term central line placement, fibrosis around pacemaker leads, thoracic outlet syndrome, and malignancy. Unfortunately, the incidence of PTS in upper DVT patients is quite high at around 30%.[87] There have been no randomized control led trials assessing the efficacy of invasive thrombolysis in preventing PTS in these patients. A trial of anticoagulation and close monitoring followed by treating the underlying causes of venous stasis in the upper extremities should form the treatment strategy in upper extremity DVT.[87] In the Catheter Study, Kovacs et al successfully treated 74 cancer patients suffering central line associated DVT with low molecular weight heparin and warfarin without the need for catheter removal.[88]

In patients with pacemakers or defibrillators, a trial of anticoagulation should be attempted prior to removing the device. For patients with no identifiable risk factors, or patients with effort thrombosis (upper extremity DVT following sporting activities), thoracic outlet syndrome should be suspected. CDT or PCMT should be attempted in these patients followed by vascular surgery referral for possible surgical intervention to decompress the thoracic veins.[87]

References

[1] Huang W, Goldberg RJ, Anderson FA, Kiefe CI, Spence FA. Secular trends in occurrence of acute venous thromboembolism: the Worcester VTE Study (1985–2009). Am J Med. 2014; 127 (9):829–83–9–.e5

[2] Cecilia Becattini C, Agnelli G, Maggioni AP, et al. Contemporary management and clinical course of acute pulmonary embolism: the cope study. Thromb Haemost. 2023; 9. Online ahead of print.

[3] Søgaard KK, Schmidt M, Pedersen L, Horváth-Puhó E, Sørensen HT. 30-year mortality after venous thromboembolism: a population-based cohort study. Circulation. 2014; 130 (10):829–836

[4] Prandoni P, Noventa F, Ghirarduzzi A, et al. The risk of recurrent venous thromboembolism after discontinuing anticoagulation in patients with acute proximal deep vein thrombosis or pulmonary embolism. A prospective cohort study in 1,626 patients. Haematologica. 2007; 92(2):199–205

[5] Kahn SR. How I treat postthrombotic syndrome. Blood. 2009; 114(21):4624–4631

[6] Kahn SR, Shrier I, Julian JA, et al. Determinants and time course of the postthrombotic syndrome after acute deep venous thrombosis. Ann Intern Med. 2008; 149(10):698–707

[7] Goldenberg NA, Donadini MP, Kahn SR, et al. Post-thrombotic syndrome in children: a systematic review of frequency of occurrence, validity of outcome measures, and prognostic factors. Haematologica. 2010; 95(11):1952–1959

[8] Kolbach DN, Neumann HA, Prins MH. Definition of the post-thrombotic syndrome, differences between existing classifications. Eur J Vasc Endovasc Surg. 2005; 30(4):404–414

[9] Kahn SR, Ginsberg JS. Relationship between deep venous thrombosis and the postthrombotic syndrome. Arch Intern Med. 2004; 164(1):17–26

[10] Vedantham S. Valvular dysfunction and venous obstruction in the post-thrombotic syndrome. Thromb Res. 2009; 123(4) Suppl 4:S62–S65

[11] Deatrick KB, Elfline M, Baker N, et al. Postthrombotic vein wall remodeling: preliminary observations. J Vasc Surg. 2011; 53(1):139–146

[12] Henke PK, Varma MR, Moaveni DK, et al. Fibrotic injury after experimental deep vein thrombosis is determined by the mechanism of thrombogenesis. Thromb Haemost. 2007; 98 (5):1045–1055

[13] Bharath V, Kahn SR, Lazo-Langner A. Genetic polymorphisms of vein wall remodeling in chronic venous disease: a narrative and systematic review. Blood. 2014; 124(8):1242–1250

[14] Vedantham S, Grassi CJ, Ferral H, et al. Technology Assessment Committee of the Society of Interventional Radiology. Reporting standards for endovascular treatment of lower extremity deep vein thrombosis. J Vasc Interv Radiol. 2006; 17 (3):417–434– Republished in: J Vasc Interv Radiol 2009;20(7 Suppl):S391–S408

[15] Ouriel K, Green RM, Greenberg RK, Clair DG. The anatomy of deep venous thrombosis of the lower extremity. J Vasc Surg. 2000; 31(5):895–900

[16] Liu J, Liu P, Xia K, Chen L, Wu X. Iliac vein compression syndrome (IVCS): an under-recognized risk factor for left-sided deep venous thrombosis (DVT) in old hip fracture patients. Med Sci Monit. 2017; 23:2078–2082

[17] Robert-Ebadi H, Righini M. Management of distal deep vein thrombosis. Thromb Res. 2017; 149:48–55

[18] Douketis JD, Crowther MA, Foster GA, Ginsberg JS. Does the location of thrombosis determine the risk of disease recurrence in patients with proximal deep vein thrombosis? Am J Med. 2001; 110(7):515–519

[19] Galanaud JP, Quenet S, Rivron-Guillot K, et al. RIETE INVESTIGATORS. Comparison of the clinical history of symptomatic isolated distal deep-vein thrombosis vs. proximal deep vein thrombosis in 11086 patients. J Thromb Haemost. 2009; 7 (12):2028–2034

[20] Kearon C, Ginsberg JS, Hirsh J. The role of venous ultrasonography in the diagnosis of suspected deep venous thrombosis and pulmonary embolism. Ann Intern Med. 1998; 129(12): 1044–1049

[21] Goodacre S, Sampson F, Thomas S, van Beek E, Sutton A. Systematic review and meta-analysis of the diagnostic accuracy of ultrasonography for deep vein thrombosis. BMC Med Imaging. 2005; 5:6

[22] Johnson SA, Stevens SM, Woller SC, et al. Risk of deep vein thrombosis following a single negative whole-leg compression ultrasound: a systematic review and meta-analysis. JAMA. 2010; 303(5):438–445

[23] Kearon C, Kahn SR, Agnelli G, Goldhaber S, Raskob GE, Comerota AJ. Antithrombotic therapy for venous thromboembolic disease: American College of Chest Physicians Evidence-Based Clinical Practice Guidelines (8th Edition). Chest. 2008; 133(6) Suppl:454S–545S– Erratum in: Chest. 2008 Oct; 134(4):892

[24] Kearon C, Akl EA, Comerota AJ, et al. Antithrombotic therapy for VTE disease: Antithrombotic Therapy and Prevention of Thrombosis, 9th ed: American College of Chest Physicians Evidence-Based Clinical Practice Guidelines. Chest. 2012;141: e419S–94S. The international guideline for treatment of venous thromboembolism.

[25] National Institute for Health and Care Excellence. Venous thromboembolic diseases: diagnosis, management and thrombophilia testing. Accessed at: https://www.nice.org.uk/ guidance/CG144. Published 2020

[26] Nicolaides AN, Fareed J, Kakkar AK, et al. Prevention and treatment of venous thromboembolism—international consensus statement. Int Angiol. 2013; 32(2):111–260

[27] Büller HR, Davidson BL, Decousus H, et al. Matisse Investigators. Fondaparinux or enoxaparin for the initial treatment of symptomatic deep venous thrombosis: a randomized trial. Ann Intern Med. 2004; 140(11):867–873

[28] Kearon C, Ginsberg JS, Julian JA, et al. Fixed-Dose Heparin (FIDO) Investigators. Comparison of fixed-dose weight-adjusted unfractionated heparin and low-molecular-weight heparin for acute treatment of venous thromboembolism. JAMA. 2006; 296(8):935–942

[29] Merli G, Spiro TE, Olsson CG, et al. Enoxaparin Clinical Trial Group. Subcutaneous enoxaparin once or twice daily compared with intravenous unfractionated heparin for treatment of venous thromboembolic disease. Ann Intern Med. 2001; 134(3):191–202

[30] Hull RD, Townshend G. Long-term treatment of deep-vein thrombosis with low-molecular-weight heparin: an update of the evidence. Thromb Haemost. 2013; 110(1):14–22

[31] Büller HR, Davidson BL, Decousus H, et al. Matisse Investigators. Subcutaneous fondaparinux versus intravenous unfractionated heparin in the initial treatment of pulmonary embolism. N Engl J Med. 2003; 349(18):1695–1702– Erratum in: N Engl J Med. 2004 Jan 22; 350(4):423

[32] Sharifi M, Bay C, Nowroozi S, Bentz S, Valeros G, Memari S. Catheter-directed thrombolysis with argatroban and tPA for massive iliac and femoropopliteal vein thrombosis. Cardiovasc Intervent Radiol. 2013; 36(6):1586–1590

[33] Brenner B, Hoffman R. Emerging options in the treatment of deep vein thrombosis and pulmonary embolism. Blood Rev. 2011; 25(5):215–221

[34] Franchini M, Mannucci PM. New anticoagulants for treatment of venous thromboembolism. Eur J Intern Med. 2012; 23(8):692–695

[35] Poulsen BK, Grove EL, Husted SE. New oral anticoagulants: a review of the literature with particular emphasis on patients with impaired renal function. Drugs. 2012; 72(13):1739–1753

[36] Becattini C, Vedovati MC, Agnelli G. Old and new oral anticoagulants for venous thromboembolism and atrial fibrillation: a review of the literature. Thromb Res. 2012; 129(3):392–400

[37] Agnelli G, Gallus A, Goldhaber SZ, et al. ODIXa-DVT Study Investigators. Treatment of proximal deep-vein thrombosis with the oral direct factor Xa inhibitor rivaroxaban (BAY 59–7939): the ODIXa-DVT (Oral Direct Factor Xa Inhibitor BAY 59–7939 in Patients With Acute Symptomatic Deep-Vein Thrombosis) study. Circulation. 2007; 116(2):180–187

[38] Buller HR, Lensing AWA, Prins MH, et al. Einstein-DVT Dose-Ranging Study investigators. A dose-ranging study evaluating once-daily oral administration of the factor Xa inhibitor rivaroxaban in the treatment of patients with acute symptomatic deep vein thrombosis: the Einstein-DVT Dose-Ranging Study. Blood. 2008; 112(6):2242–2247

[39] Eriksson BI, Borris LC, Friedman RJ, et al. RECORD1 Study Group. Rivaroxaban versus enoxaparin for thromboprophylaxis after hip arthroplasty. N Engl J Med. 2008; 358(26): 2765–2775

[40] Kakkar AK, Brenner B, Dahl OE, et al. RECORD2 Investigators. Extended duration rivaroxaban versus short-term enoxaparin for the prevention of venous thromboembolism after total

hip arthroplasty: a double-blind, randomised controlled trial. Lancet. 2008; 372(9632):31–39

[41] Agnelli G, Buller HR, Cohen A, et al. AMPLIFY Investigators. Oral apixaban for the treatment of acute venous thromboembolism. N Engl J Med. 2013; 369(9):799–808

[42] Raskob G, Büller H, Prins M, et al. Hokusai-VTE Investigators. Edoxaban for the long-term treatment of venous thromboembolism: rationale and design of the Hokusai-venous thromboembolism study—methodological implications for clinical trials. J Thromb Haemost. 2013; 11(7):1287–1294

[43] Schulman S, Kearon C, Kakkar AK, et al. RE-COVER Study Group. Dabigatran versus warfarin in the treatment of acute venous thromboembolism. N Engl J Med. 2009; 361(24): 2342–2352

[44] Schulman S, Kearon C, Kakkar AK, et al. RE-MEDY Trial Investigators, RE-SONATE Trial Investigators. Extended use of dabigatran, warfarin, or placebo in venous thromboembolism. N Engl J Med. 2013; 368(8):709–718

[45] Eriksson BI, Dahl OE, Rosencher N, et al. RE-NOVATE Study Group. Dabigatran etexilate versus enoxaparin for prevention of venous thromboembolism after total hip replacement: a randomised, double-blind, non-inferiority trial. Lancet. 2007; 370(9591):949–956

[46] Lassen MR, Ageno W, Borris LC, et al. RECORD3 Investigators. Rivaroxaban versus enoxaparin for thromboprophylaxis after total knee arthroplasty. N Engl J Med. 2008; 358 (26):2776–2786

[47] Lassen MR, Gallus A, Raskob GE, Pineo G, Chen D, Ramirez LM, ADVANCE-3 Investigators. Apixaban versus enoxaparin for thromboprophylaxis after hip replacement. N Engl J Med. 2010; 363(26):2487–2498

[48] Friedman RJ, Dahl OE, Rosencher N, et al. RE-MOBILIZE, RE-MODEL, RE-NOVATE Steering Committees. Dabigatran versus enoxaparin for prevention of venous thromboembolism after hip or knee arthroplasty: a pooled analysis of three trials. Thromb Res. 2010; 126(3):175–182

[49] Haig Y, Enden T, Slagsvold CE, Sandvik L, Sandset PM, Kløw NE. Determinants of early and long-term efficacy of catheter-directed thrombolysis in proximal deep vein thrombosis. J Vasc Interv Radiol. 2013; 24(1):17–24, quiz 26

[50] Patel NH, Plorde JJ, Meissner M. Catheter-directed thrombolysis in the treatment of phlegmasia cerulea dolens. Ann Vasc Surg. 1998; 12(5):471–475

[51] Vedantham S, Sista AK, Klein SJ, et al. Society of Interventional Radiology and Cardiovascular and Interventional Radiological Society of Europe Standards of Practice Committees. Quality improvement guidelines for the treatment of lower-extremity deep vein thrombosis with use of endovascular thrombus removal. J Vasc Interv Radiol. 2014; 25 (9):1317–1325

[52] Kahn SR, Shbaklo H, Lamping DL, et al. Determinants of health-related quality of life during the 2 years following deep vein thrombosis. J Thromb Haemost. 2008; 6(7):1105–1112

[53] Elliot MS, Immelman EJ, Jeffery P, et al. A comparative randomized trial of heparin versus streptokinase in the treatment of acute proximal venous thrombosis: an interim report of a prospective trial. Br J Surg. 1979; 66(12):838–843

[54] Arnesen H, Høiseth A, Ly B. Streptokinase of heparin in the treatment of deep vein thrombosis. Follow-up results of a prospective study. Acta Med Scand. 1982; 211(1–2):65–68

[55] Goldhaber SZ, Buring JE, Lipnick RJ, Hennekens CH. Pooled analyses of randomized trials of streptokinase and heparin in phlebographically documented acute deep venous thrombosis. Am J Med. 1984; 76(3):393–397

[56] Turpie AGG, Levine MN, Hirsh J, et al. Tissue plasminogen activator (rt-PA) vs heparin in deep vein thrombosis. Results of a randomized trial. Chest. 1990; 97(4) Suppl:172S–175S

[57] Goldhaber SZ, Meyerovitz MF, Green D, et al. Randomized controlled trial of tissue plasminogen activator in proximal deep venous thrombosis. Am J Med. 1990; 88(3):235–240

[58] Schwieder G, Grimm W, Siemens HJ, et al. Intermittent regional therapy with rt-PA is not superior to systemic thrombolysis in deep vein thrombosis (DVT)—a German multicenter trial. Thromb Haemost. 1995; 74(5):1240–1243

[59] Lu T, Loh TM, El-Sayed HF, Davies MG. Single-center retrospective review of ultrasound-accelerated versus traditional catheter-directed thrombolysis for acute lower extremity deep venous thrombosis. Vascular. 2017; 25(5):525–532

[60] Foegh P, Jensen LP, Klitfod L, Broholm R, Bækgaard N. Editor's choice—factors associated with long-term outcome in 191 patients with ilio-femoral DVT treated with catheter-directed thrombolysis. Eur J Vasc Endovasc Surg. 2017; 53(3): 419–424

[61] Okrent D, Messersmith R, Buckman J. Transcatheter fibrinolytic therapy and angioplasty for left iliofemoral venous thrombosis. J Vasc Interv Radiol. 1991; 2(2):195–197, discussion 198–200

[62] Molina JE, Hunter DW, Yedlicka JW, Cerra FB. Thrombolytic therapy for postoperative pulmonary embolism. Am J Surg. 1992; 163(4):375–380, discussion 380–381

[63] Semba CP, Dake MD. Iliofemoral deep venous thrombosis: aggressive therapy with catheter-directed thrombolysis. Radiology. 1994; 191(2):487–494

[64] Bjarnason H, Kruse JR, Asinger DA, et al. Iliofemoral deep venous thrombosis: safety and efficacy outcome during 5 years of catheter-directed thrombolytic therapy. J Vasc Interv Radiol. 1997; 8(3):405–418

[65] Mewissen MW, Seabrook GR, Meissner MH, Cynamon J, Labropoulos N, Haughton SH. Catheter-directed thrombolysis for lower extremity deep venous thrombosis: report of a national multicenter registry. Radiology. 1999; 211(1):39–49

[66] Elsharawy M, Elzayat E. Early results of thrombolysis vs anticoagulation in iliofemoral venous thrombosis. A randomised clinical trial. Eur J Vasc Endovasc Surg. 2002; 24(3):209–214

[67] Haig Y, Enden T, Grøtta O, et al. Post-thrombotic syndrome after catheter-directed thrombolysis for deep vein thrombosis (CaVenT): 5-year follow-up results of an open-label, randomised controlled trial. Lancet Haematol. 2016;3(2): e64–71

[68] Vedantham S, Goldhaber SZ, Julian JA, Kahn SR, Jaff MR, Cohen DJ, Magnuson E, Razavi MK, Comerota AJ, Gornik HL, et al. Pharmacomechanical catheter-directed thrombolysis for deep-vein thrombosis. N Engl J Med. 2017;377:2240–2252

[69] Kim HS, Patra A, Paxton BE, Khan J, Streiff MB. Adjunctive percutaneous mechanical thrombectomy for lower-extremity deep vein thrombosis: clinical and economic outcomes. J Vasc Interv Radiol. 2006; 17(7):1099–1104

[70] Notten P, Ten Cate-Hoek AJ, Arnoldussen C, Strijkers RH, de Smet A, Tick LW, van de Poel MH, Wikkeling OR, Vleming LJ, Koster A, et al. Ultrasound-accelerated catheter-directed thrombolysis versus anticoagulation for the prevention of post-thrombotic syndrome (CAVA): a single-blind, multicentre, randomised trial. Lancet Haematol. 2020;7:e40–e49

[71] Lin PH, Zhou W, Dardik A, et al. Catheter-direct thrombolysis versus pharmacomechanical thrombectomy for treatment of symptomatic lower extremity deep venous thrombosis. Am J Surg. 2006; 192(6):782–788

[72] Enden T, Resch S, White C, Wik HS, Kløw NE, Sandset PM. Cost-effectiveness of additional catheter-directed thrombolysis

for deep vein thrombosis. J Thromb Haemost. 2013; 11(6): 1032–1042

[73] Sugimoto K, Hofmann LV, Razavi MK, et al. The safety, efficacy, and pharmacoeconomics of low-dose alteplase compared with urokinase for catheter-directed thrombolysis of arterial and venous occlusions. J Vasc Surg. 2003; 37(3):512–517

[74] Razavi MK, Wong H, Kee ST, Sze DY, Semba CP, Dake MD. Initial clinical results of tenecteplase (TNK) in catheter-directed thrombolytic therapy. J Endovasc Ther. 2002; 9(5):593–598

[75] Srinivas BC, Patra S, Nagesh CM, Reddy B, Manjunath CN. Catheter-directed thrombolysis along with mechanical thromboaspiration versus anticoagulation alone in the management of lower limb deep venous thrombosis—a comparative study. Int J Angiol. 2014; 23(4):247–254

[76] Cynamon J, Stein EG, Dym RJ, Jagust MB, Binkert CA, Baum RA. A new method for aggressive management of deep vein thrombosis: retrospective study of the power pulse technique. J Vasc Interv Radiol. 2006; 17(6):1043–1049

[77] Weissler EH, Cox MW, Commander SJ, Williams ZF. Restoring Venous Patency with the ClotTriever Following Deep Vein Thrombosis. Ann Vasc Surg. 2023; 88:268–273

[78] Garcia MJ, Lookstein R, Malhotra R, et al. Endovascular management of deep vein thrombosis with rheolytic thrombectomy: final report of the Prospective Multicenter PEARL (Peripheral Use of AngioJet Rheolytic Thrombectomy with a Variety of Catheter Lengths) registry. J Vasc Interv Radiol. 2015; 26(6):777–785, quiz 786

[79] Sharifi M, Mehdipour M, Bay C, Smith G, Sharifi J. Endovenous therapy for deep venous thrombosis: the TORPEDO trial. Catheter Cardiovasc Interv. 2010; 76(3):316–325

[80] Vedantham S, Goldhaber SZ, Kahn SR, et al. Rationale and design of the ATTRACT Study: a multicenter randomized trial to evaluate pharmacomechanical catheter-directed thrombolysis for the prevention of postthrombotic syndrome in patients with proximal deep vein thrombosis. Am Heart J. 2013; 165(4):523–530.e3

[81] Kearon C, Akl EA, Ornelas J, et al. Antithrombotic therapy for VTE disease: CHEST Guideline and Expert Panel Report. Chest. 2016; 149(2):315–352

[82] Jaff MR, McMurtry MS, Archer SL, et al. American Heart Association Council on Cardiopulmonary, Critical Care, Perioperative and Resuscitation, American Heart Association Council on Peripheral Vascular Disease, American Heart Association Council on Arteriosclerosis, Thrombosis and Vascular Biology. Management of massive and submassive pulmonary embolism, iliofemoral deep vein thrombosis, and chronic thromboembolic pulmonary hypertension: a scientific statement from the American Heart Association. Circulation. 2011; 123 (16):1788–1830

[83] Liu G, Liu X, Wang R, et al. Catheter-directed thrombolysis of acute entire limb deep vein thrombosis from below the knee access: a retrospective analysis of a single-center experience. Catheter Cardiovasc Interv. 2018; 91(2):310–317

[84] Patel NH, Stookey KR, Ketcham DB, Cragg AH. Endovascular management of acute extensive iliofemoral deep venous thrombosis caused by May-Thurner syndrome. J Vasc Interv Radiol. 2000; 11(10):1297–1302

[85] Wakefield TW, Myers DD, Henke PK. Role of selectins and fibrinolysis in VTE. Thromb Res. 2009; 123 Suppl 4:S35–S40

[86] Isma N, Svensson PJ, Gottsäter A, Lindblad B. Upper extremity deep venous thrombosis in the population-based Malmö thrombophilia study (MATS). Epidemiology, risk factors, recurrence risk, and mortality. Thromb Res. 2010; 125(6):e335–e338

[87] Vazquez FJ, Paulin P, Poodts D, Gándara E. Preferred management of primary deep arm thrombosis. Eur J Vasc Endovasc Surg. 2017; 53(5):744–751

[88] Kovacs MJ, Kahn SR, Rodger M, et al. A pilot study of central venous catheter survival in cancer patients using low-molecular-weight heparin (dalteparin) and warfarin without catheter removal for the treatment of upper extremity deep vein thrombosis (The Catheter Study). J Thromb Haemost. 2007; 5(8):1650–1653

Chapter 5

Inferior Vena Cava Filter Placement

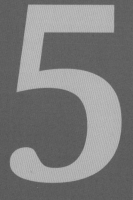

5 Inferior Vena Cava Filter Placement

David Heister and Thomas B. Kinney

keyword: IVC filter

5.1 Introduction

It has been estimated that between 350,000 and 500,000 individuals are affected by deep venous thrombosis and pulmonary embolism (DVT/PE) each year in America with a large proportion of those patients needing inpatient management for new and recurrent DVT/PE, also defined as venous thromboembolism (VTE). This disease process is conservatively estimated to cost the U.S. medical system 7 to 10 billion dollars annually.[1] Additionally, U.S. PE mortality has been estimated at 50,000 to 100,000 people annually, and is one of the leading causes of preventable inpatient mortality.[2]

While the primary management of VTE is pharmacologic, inferior vena cava (IVC) filters can provide an important additional mechanism for the protection of patients from PE. Due a combination of factors, the number of filter insertions rose rapidly between 1998 and 2008.[3]

The goal of IVC filter placement is the prevention of clinically significant and/or fatal PE. While IVC filters have been shown to reduce the risk of PE in randomized trials, they have also been found to increase the risk of DVT and have not been shown to improve overall mortality.[4] There are currently a variety of clinical indications for IVC filter placement. Some of these indications have a fair amount of supporting data and support from associated medical society. Other filter placement indications may be justified but have substantially fewer supporting data. Consequently, the interventionalists must be aware of the various filter designs, filter indications, the strength of the evidence behind these indications, and the associated risk factors in order to make a well-informed management decision for their patient.

5.2 History and Background of IVC Filters

It has long been understood that lower extremity thrombus can result in PE. Bottini was the first to perform a caval ligation to prevent PE in 1893.

In 1967, the first IVC filter was released (Mobin-Uddin). The original Greenfield filter was released in 1973. In 1984, the techniques for percutaneous insertion were first described. The first retrievable filter was approved by the Food and Drug Administration (FDA) in 2003. Multiple designs have subsequently been developed, and the number of filters deployed and the use over last 30 to 40 years has continued to rise rapidly. IVC filter use started to decline in 2010, which coincided with an FDA warning to remove filters when no longer needed.

There are four overall classes of IVC filters. Permanent filters were the first to receive FDA approval and subsequently have the greatest amount of longitudinal data. Retrievable (optional) filters are devices that may remain permanently, but may also be retrieved depending on the clinical situation. Convertible filters are permanent devices that can be altered to no longer function as filters (i.e., they can be converted from a filter to a permanent caval stent). The last type of filter is the temporary filter, which is appropriately approved for short-term usage only.

5.3 IVC Filter Placement Indications

IVC filters are designed to prevent large venous embolic phenomena originating from the legs and pelvis from entering the lungs. The primary means of VTE therapy and prophylaxis are pharmacologic, and prior epidemiological studies into VTE have found that approximately 90% of VTE disease is treated with anticoagulation alone,[5] but IVC filters are indicated in a significant minority of patients with VTE.

The PREPIC (Prévention du Risque d'Embolie Pulmonaire par Interruption Cave) study is one of the highest quality and one of the most frequently cited studies investigating the efficacy of IVC filters. PREPIC was a randomized, multicenter study conducted on 400 patients with acute proximal DVT. Participants were randomized to receive anticoagulation or anticoagulation plus an IVC filter. The data demonstrated a significant decrease in pulmonary emboli in the filter group in both the acute and chronic settings (12 days and 2 years). Follow-up studies found that at 8 years, vena cava filters reduced the risk of PE but increased the risk of DVT and had no effect on overall mortality.[4,6] The PREPIC II study found that IVC filter placement did not reduce the risk of symptomatic PE as compared to anticoagulation alone.[7] These studies and other retrospective and population-based studies have formed the basis of several medical societies' statement papers that provide guidelines to assist in defining appropriate indications for IVC filter placement (e.g., American College of Chest Physicians [ACCP], American College of Radiology [ACR], American Heart Association [AHA], Eastern Association for the Surgery of Trauma [EAST], Society for Interventional Radiology [SIR]).[8,9,10,11,12]

The SIR guidelines are largely directed toward identifying the presence and extent of VTE burden and the effectiveness of primary prophylaxis (i.e., anticoagulation).[8] Classic (absolute) indications all occur in the setting of proven VTE and include recurrent VTE despite anticoagulation (anticoagulation failure), contraindications to anticoagulation,

complications to anticoagulation, and inability to achieve/maintain therapeutic anticoagulation. Relative or expanded indications for IVC filter placement also occur in the setting of known VTE but in clinical situations where there may be a reasonable expectation of benefit but the value of IVC filtration continues to be debated. These relative/expanded indications include large VTE burden (iliocaval DVT or large free-floating proximal DVT), difficulty establishing therapeutic anticoagulation, chronic thromboembolic disease with thromboendarterectomy, iliocaval thrombus thrombolysis, poor compliance with anticoagulation, recurrent PE with filter (possibly compromised) in place, the patient being a poor candidate for anticoagulation (e.g., a patient with a history of multiple falls), and patients with concern for a possible complication from anticoagulation (▶ Table 5.1).

The last class of IVC filter indications are the prophylactic filters, which are placed in the absence of known VTE, but in the setting of high

Table 5.1 Classic, extended, and prophylactic indications for IVC filter placement

Patients with documented VTE and classic indications	Patients with documented VTE and expanded indications	Patients without VTE
Contraindication to anticoagulation	Iliocaval or large free-floating proximal DVT	Trauma patient with high risk of VTE
Complication of anticoagulation necessitating cessation	Inability to achieve/maintain adequate anticoagulation	Surgical procedure in a patient at high risk of VTE
Failure of anticoagulation	Massive PE with residual DVT in a patient at risk of further PE	Medical condition with high risk of VTE
Propagation/progression of DVT during therapeutic anticoagulation	Chronic venous thromboembolism treated with thromboendarterectomy	
	Thrombolysis of iliocaval DVT	
	VTE with limited cardiopulmonary reserve	
	Recurrent PE with IVC filter in place (filter failure)	
	Poor compliance with anticoagulation	
	High risk of complication of anticoagulation (e.g., high fall risk)	

Abbreviations: DVT, deep venous thrombosis; IVC, inferior vena cava; PE, pulmonary embolism; VTE, venous thromboembolism.
Source: DeYoung E, Minocha J. Inferior vena cava filters: guidelines, best practice, and expanding indications. Semin Intervent Radiol 2016;33(2):65–70.

clinical risk of PE. The average incidence of DVT in the general trauma population is 42% (ranging from 18 to 90%) and the reported incidence of PE in patients with spinal cord injury is 10% (range: 4–22%). Many of these patients also have contraindications to anticoagulation and thus some groups have recommended IVC filtration as a logical step to reduce the incidence of clinically significant PE. Prophylactic filters have also been considered in surgical (e.g., bariatric surgery) and medical (e.g., malignancy) situations.[11,13]

Due to a lack of high-quality data, debate persists as to exactly which patients should receive prophylactic IVC filters. For example, the EAST released guidelines in 2002 indicating IVC filtration should be considered in immobilized patients at high risk of a DVT/PE who cannot be anticoagulated.[11] Although they also cite a lack of strong evidence and list this as a "level 3" recommendation. On the contrary, the ACCP guidelines do not recommend for the placement of prophylactic IVC filters.[14] If a prophylactic filter is placed, it is a priority to reevaluate the patient daily for the possibility of restarting primary prophylaxis and removing the filter as soon as possible.[8] As described in the SIR guidelines, these recommendations are derived by consensus and are meant to be used as "suggestions" and should always be adopted to local practices.

5.4 Contraindications

Previously documented contraindications to IVC filter placement are listed as a lack of access route to the vena cava or lack of adequate space in the IVC for placement of filter.[8] Severe and uncorrectable coagulopathy and bacteremia are relative contraindications, which have been debated in the literature.[15] There have been rare reports of metal allergies (mostly silver).

Filter terminology/complications: Pulmonary emboli are known to occur despite the placement of IVC filters, and no studies have conclusively shown that one design of IVC filter is superior to the others in terms of PE preventions (▶ Table 5.2). Most commonly used filters have been found to have similar efficacy in preventing PE.

However, different filter designs have been found to be prone to various different complications. Early complications include access site complications, insertional problems (filter malfunction, tilt > 15 degrees), malposition, and filter migration. Delayed complications include caval thrombosis, caval perforation, filter fracture, recurrent PE, and filter migration.

The SIR has formulated definitions for several potential IVC filter complications.

Insertion problems refer to malfunctions of the filter or deployment system such as incomplete filter opening or filter tilt more than 15 degrees from the IVC axis. Placement of the filter outside of the target zone (e.g., infrarenal IVC) will also be considered an insertional problem. The presence of an occluding thrombus in the IVC after filter insertion is defined as IVC thrombotic occlusion. IVC penetration is defined as filter strut or anchor devices extending more than 3 mm outside the wall of the IVC. Filter movement is a change in filter position of more than 2 cm as compared

Table 5.2 Filter characteristic

	Caval patency (%)	Recurrent PE (%)	Introducer size (OD), Fr	Carrier size (Fr)
24FSGF	96	4	29	24
OTWSGF	95	N/A	15	12
TGF	91–99	3–4	14	12
BNF	81–97	3–4	14	11
VTF	67–92	3.5	13	10
SNF	92	1.1	9	7

Abbreviations: OD, outer diameter; PE, pulmonary embolism; OTWSFG, Over-the-Wire Stainless Steel Greenfield Filter; TGF, Titanium Greenfield Filter; BNF, Bird's Nest Filter; SNF, Simon Nitinol Filter; VTF, Vena-Tech Filter; SGF, Stainless Steel Greenfield Filter.
Source: Namyslowski J. Vena Cava Filters. *Seminars in Interventional Radiology* 2001; 18(02): 119–130.

with its original deployment position. Filter embolization is postdeployment movement of the filter or its components to a distant anatomical site. Filter fracture is any loss of a filter's structural integrity (i.e., breakage or separation of filter). Occlusive or nonocclusive thrombus developing at the venotomy site after filter insertion is defined as access site thrombus. These may also include arteriovenous fistula, hematoma, or bleeding requiring a transfusion.[15]

The SIR has also published guidelines with reported rates of IVC filter complications with associated thresholds (▶ Table 5.3).

5.5 Choosing a Filter

There are many characteristics of an ideal IVC filter. It should provide adequate filtration without significantly limiting flow. It should be nonthrombogenic, biocompatible, and have an infinite implant life. Fixation should be secured with no migration or tilting. It would have ease of percutaneous insertion with a small delivery system and the release mechanism should be easy to use. Additionally, it will be potentially amenable to repositioning, and magnetic resonance imaging compatible. It would have a low cost, and low access site thrombosis.

Many design shapes have been developed to meet these goals, including conical, conical with an umbrella, conical with an associated cylinder, biconical with a cylinder, and complex ▶ Fig. 5.1.[16] Each design/product has more or less of each of these competing characteristics, and this likely explains why there is an abundance of product designs without any showing clear superiority to the rest.[8] However, different designs have been found to be more or less prone to a variety of complications including fracture, filter tilting, IVC perforation, and migration. As a result, it is important to be familiar with the limitations of each filter and also to consider each patient's clinical situation when choosing a filter.

For example, a prophylactically placed filter may never develop a DVT or subject the filter to a clot

Table 5.3 Reported rates of complications and adverse events involving the inferior vena cava filters

Complication	Reported rate (%)
IVC penetration	0–41
IVC occlusion	2–30
Access site thrombosis	0–25
Insertion complication	5–23
Filter migration	0–18
Filter fracture	2–10
IVC filter deployment outside of target region	1–9
Recurrent PE	0.5–6
Filter embolization	< 1
Death	0.12

Abbreviations: IVC, inferior vena cava; PE, pulmonary embolism.
Source: *Namyslowski J. Vena cava filters. Semin Intervent Radiol. 2015;32(01):034–041.*

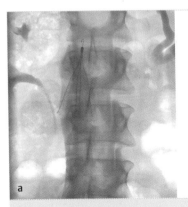
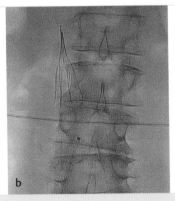
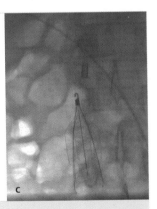

Fig. 5.1 Examples of commercially available IVC filters, including **(a)** Cook Günther Tulip; **(b)** Argon Option; and **(c)** Bard Denali IVC filters.

challenge. This prophylactic filter will ideally be removed before long-term complications will be a concern. As a result, long-term follow-up data may be less of a priority than ensuring a minimal risk profile of deployment and retrieval. On the contrary, patients with an indication for a permanent filter may have an increased risk of long-term complications of IVC filter placement, and it may be worth considering placing a filter with more long-term safety data.

5.5.1 Permanent and Removable Filters

When choosing an IVC filter for deployment, a major decision to consider is whether to place a permanent or a removable (optional) IVC filter. Permanent filters are indicated in some clinical indications, but retrievable filters have previously been defined as permanent devices designed for image-guided percutaneous removal during device-specific time windows.[8] Removable filters may be placed with the intent for removal but becomes "permanent" once it is deemed that filter removal is no longer indicated.

While the SIR guidelines state that there are no unique indications for removable filters that are distinct from permanent filters, if the clinical scenario requires permanent IVC filtration, it may be reasonable to place a filter with the largest long-term safety data. While permanent filters do have more historical safety data, and as a group permanent, filters have been shown to have less reported complications.[17] Many of the reported complications have been generated from a few retrievable filter styles that have subsequently been recalled. Thus, it is possible that this difference in complication rates has more to do with device-specific product design and less to do with each device's listing as permanent or retrievable.

The decision to place a retrievable filter is typically based on the expectation that the patient's situation of increased VTE risk/burden and/or limitations of administering primary VTE prophylaxis is limited in duration. In 2010 and again in 2014, the FDA issued a statement encouraging clinicians to remove IVC filters as soon as protection for PE is no longer needed.[18] Many contraindications to anticoagulation (e.g., bleeding) are temporary, and once the period of contraindication passes, patients again become candidates for anticoagulation, which negates the need for IVC

filtration. At this time, consideration can begin for removal of the filter.[8]

A recent review summarized the reports of device-specific complications from multiple evidence-based electronic resources and compiled the figures presented in ▶ Table 5.4. It was noted that conical filters (e.g., Bard Recovery/G2 or Cook Günther Tulip) were more prone to IVC penetration, whereas cylindrical filters (e.g., Vena-Tech, TrapEase, and OptEase) were more associated with caval thrombosis.

5.6 Deployment Methods

IVC filters are now typically placed percutaneously either from the right common femoral vein or from the right internal jugular vein, although alternate access sites have been described (e.g., left sided or even via the antecubital vein).

Venography is typically used to define caval anatomy. Particularly relevant findings on the cavogram include the size of the vena cava, presence of thrombus, bilateral iliac inflow, identification of renal vein inflow, and angulation of the IVC. Venography is important to exclude the presence of caval variants (e.g., caval duplication, left-sided cava, and circumaortic renal veins) that can also be present. A variety of additional techniques have been described including the use of bedside fluoroscopy to place filter, using CO_2 as the contrast agent, intravascular ultrasound (US) guided filter placement, and even abdominal US-guided placement. Due to the widespread use of imaging, many patients with an indication for an IVC filter will have previous axial imaging that should be used to evaluate the IVC anatomy prior to starting the procedure.

5.6.1 Placement Location

IVC filters are typically placed in the infrarenal IVC with the apex just below the lowest renal vein (▶ Fig. 5.2). This location provides a stable section of vessel that has adequate inflow from the renal veins and is less likely to be affected by respiratory and cardiac motion present in the suprarenal IVC; additionally, formation of IVC thrombus typically extends caudally and is less likely to affect renal perfusion.

Suprarenal filters can also be indicated in certain situations. For example: occluded infrarenal cava, duplicated IVC, and large thrombus burden present in a renal or gonadal vein or even in a

Table 5.4 Highest reported radiographically identifiable complications for each filter type

Device (year FDA cleared)	Fracture	IVC perforation	Migration	IVC occlusion
ALN (2008)	Case reports (0%)	3.4% (3.4%)	3% (1.4–3%)	Case reports (0%)
Recovery (2003/2005[a])	39.5% at 65.7 mo 25% (5.5–25%)	100% (27–100%)	10% (0–10%)	Case reports (0%)
G2 (2005/2008[a]) G2X (2008) Eclipse (2008) Meridian (2011)	38% at 60 mo 12% (1.2–12%)	44% (18–44%)	25% (12–25%)	2.2% (0–2.2%)
Denali (2013)	Case reports	2.5% (2.5%)	Limited data	Limited data
Simon Nitinol (1990)	16% (10–16%)	95% (25–95%)	5% (0–5%)	50% (3.5–50%)
LGM/Vena Tech LCM (1989)	Case reports	Case reports (0%)	18.4% (6–18.4%)	65% at 9 y (3.7%/y)
Vena Tech LP (2001)	Limited data	Case reports (0%)	Case reports (0%)	Limited data
24F SS Greenfield (1973)	Case reports	15% (2–15%)	2% (2%)	5% (2–5%)
12F SS Greenfield (1995)	0.3% (0.3%)	1% (1%)	2.6% (2.6%)	12% (5–12%)
Titanium Greenfield (1989)	3.8% (3.8%)	50%	15% (7.5–15%)	20% (3.5–20%)
Günther Tulip (2000/2003[a])	0.3% (0.3%)	78% (22–78%)	12.5% (2.4–12.5%)	4.1% (2.4–4.1%)
Celect (2007/2008[a]) Celect Platinum (2012)	5.6% (4.3–5.6%)	93% (22–93%)	4.3% (0–4.3%)	2.5% (2.5%)
Bird's Nest (1989)	4% (3–4%)	85% (85%)	1.1% (1.1%)	4.7% (2.9–4.7%)
OptEase (2002/2004[a]) TrapEase (2000)	50% (0–50%)	Case reports (0%)	0.9% (0–0.9%)	29% (0.8–29%)
Option (2009)	Limited data	10% (2.9–10%)	2% (2%)	4% (4%)
Crux (2012)	Limited data (0%)	Limited data	Limited data (0%)	Limited data (7.2% nonocclpsive IVC thrombus)

Abbreviations: FDA, Food and Drug Administration; IVC, inferior vena cava.
[a]Subsequent year when filter was cleared for retrieval indication.
Source: *Deso SE, Idakoji IA, Kuo WT. Evidence-Based Evaluation of Inferior Vena Cava Filter Complications Based on Filter Type. Semin Intervent Radiol. 2016 Jun;33(2):93–100.*

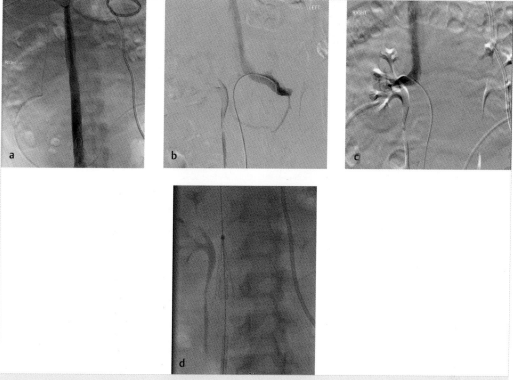

Fig. 5.2 (a) Inferior vena cavogram; **(b)** left renal venogram; and **(c)** right renal venogram prior to IVC filter placement. **(d)** Fluoroscopic image IVC filter after placement.

patient that may become pregnant. These indications must be weighed against concerns that suprarenal filters may be subjected to increased respiratory/cardiac motion (possibly making fracture, migration, and embolization more likely), caval thrombosis may extend into the renal veins and affect renal perfusion, and caval perforation in the suprarenal IVC may be more clinically significant than caval perforation in the infrarenal IVC.

5.6.2 Variants

The IVC is known to have multiple variants, and it is important to evaluate for these variants with any preprocedural axial imaging as well as during intraprocedural venography.

A megacava is defined as an IVC greater than 28 to 30 mm in the anteroposterior (AP) projection. It is estimated that 2.5 % of the population has a megacava. While the Argon Option Elite, the Cook Gunther-Tulip, and Cordis OptEase/TrapEase are approved for IVCs up to 30 mm, most IVC filters are approved for IVCs up to 28 mm. The Cook Bird's Nest is approved for an IVC up to 40 mm. Deployments of a Bird's Nest filter and bilateral iliac filters are both options in the setting of a megacava. Additional important caval variants include duplicated IVC (▶ Fig. 5.3), left-sided IVC, azygous continuation of IVC, and circumaortic renal veins.

5.7 Deployment Complications

While technical success of IVC filter deployment is expected to be greater than 97% by the SIR guidelines, deployment failures can have many origins, including incorrect caval sizing leading to filter embolization, incorrect alignment, incorrect deployment location, and incorrect orientation.[15] ▶ Fig. 5.4 demonstrates the importance of technique to confirm that a filter is adequately placed in the appropriate location.

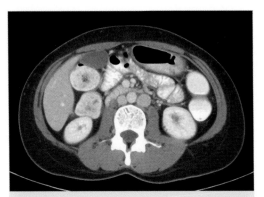

Fig. 5.3 Computed tomography (CT) of the abdomen demonstrating a duplicated IVC.

5.8 Timing of IVC Filter Placement

As is true with much of IVC filter deployment, there are insufficient data to make firm recommendations regarding the timing of filter placement, but an earlier work has attempted to separate IVC filter indications into emergent, urgent, and elective indications.[19]

This work listed emergent filter placement in patients with large VTE burden (e.g., acute PE or free-floating iliofemoral DVT) and a contraindication to anticoagulation or anticoagulation failure. Additionally, patients with large VTE burden and severely limited cardiopulmonary reserve have an indication of emergent IVC filter placement as they may be unable to tolerate any/additional embolic insults. In this setting, it was recommended that filter placement be done within the first 12 to 24 hours.

Patients with proximal DVT (popliteal and above) or with enlarging distal DVT and a contraindication to anticoagulation have a classic indication for IVC filter placement that was considered urgent, and filter deployment is recommended between 24 and 48 hours, or sooner if possible. Elective IVC filter indications are considered for patients without a current DVT but with a high risk of developing PE and/or DVT, such as elective orthopaedic surgery, or chronic thromboembolic pulmonary hypertensive patients prior to pulmonary thromboendarterectomy.

5.9 Postplacement Management

In a patient who receives an IVC filter due to an inability to anticoagulate, the patient should be constantly reevaluated for the potential to start

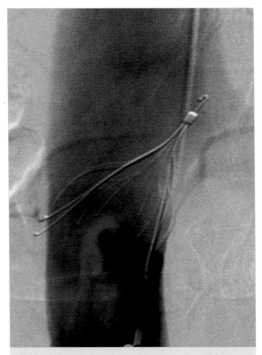

Fig. 5.4 Incorrect alignment/tilt of a Cook Celect IVC filter.

anticoagulation. That is, placement of an IVC filter does not typically change the need or timing of restarting anticoagulation.

As stated in the SIR guidelines, placement of retrievable IVC filters requires tracking and routine follow-up.[8] The decision to remove the filter or leave it as a permanent filter is often dependent on the patient's conditions and clinical events occurring after filter deployment. Prior groups have shown that retrieval rates can be substantially improved with the implementation of an IVC filter retrieval program.[20] Their data indicated that a substantial number of filters were being made permanent due to loss to follow-up and that a structured system to track and manage these patients was effective in improving successful retrieval rates. It is recommended that IVC filter deployment be tracked at a department or institutional level, and every effort for filter removal be carried out as soon as it is clinically feasible.

5.10 Conclusion

As stated in the ACCP guidelines, "Risk stratification for venous thromboembolism is challenging but essential and requires consideration of both patient and procedure-specific risk factors."[2] IVC filter deployment is an important component of the management of VTE, but the risks and benefits are not fully known, and this can make clinical decision-making difficult. It is important to remember that the 8-year follow-up data for the PREPIC study found IVC filters decreased the risk of PE, but increased the risk of DVT, and were not shown to have any mortality benefit.[4] It is important for further research to continue to investigate the optimal indications and contraindications for filter placement. Furthermore, when device-related complications do occur, the interventionalist is encouraged to report these events to the MAUDE (Manufacturer and User Facility Device Experience; www.fda.gov) database.

There are a variety of considerations when placing an IVC filter, but the interventionalist with a thorough understanding of the disease process, the patient, the procedure, and the implanted device will be equipped to make the best clinical decision.

References

[1] Grosse SD, Nelson RE, Nyarko KA, Richardson LC, Raskob GE. The economic burden of incident venous thromboembolism in the United States: a review of estimated attributable healthcare costs. Thromb Res. 2016; 137:3–10

[2] Gould MK, Garcia DA, Wren SM, et al. Prevention of VTE in nonorthopedic surgical patients. Antithrombotic Therapy and Prevention of Thrombosis, 9th ed: American College of Chest Physicians Evidence-Based Clinical Practice Guidelines. Chest. 2012; 141(2) Suppl:e227S–e277S

[3] Duszak R, Jr, Parker L, Levin DC, Rao VM. Placement and removal of inferior vena cava filters: national trends in the Medicare population. J Am Coll Radiol. 2011; 8(7):483–489

[4] PREPIC Study Group. Eight-year follow-up of patients with permanent vena cava filters in the prevention of pulmonary embolism: the PREPIC (Prévention du Risque d'Embolie Pulmonaire par Interruption Cave) randomized study. Circulation. 2005; 112:416–423

[5] Ferrari E, Baudouy M, Cerboni P, et al. Clinical epidemiology of venous thromboembolic disease. Results of a French multicentre registry. Eur Heart J. 1997; 18(4):685–691

[6] Decousus H, Leizorovicz A, Parent F, et al. A clinical trial of vena caval filters in the prevention of pulmonary embolism in patients with proximal deep-vein thrombosis. Prévention du Risque d'Embolie Pulmonaire par Interruption Cave Study Group. N Engl J Med. 1998; 338(7):409–415

[7] Mismetti P, Laporte S, Pellerin O, et al. PREPIC2 Study Group. Effect of a retrievable inferior vena cava filter plus anticoagulation vs anticoagulation alone on risk of recurrent pulmonary embolism: a randomized clinical trial. JAMA. 2015; 313 (16):1627–1635

[8] Kaufman JA, Kinney TB, Streiff MB, et al. Guidelines for the use of retrievable and convertible vena cava filters: report from the Society of Interventional Radiology multidisciplinary consensus conference. J Vasc Interv Radiol. 2006; 17(3): 449–459

[9] Kinney TB, Aryafar H, Ray CE Jr, et al; Expert Panel on Interventional Radiology. ACR Appropriateness Criteria Radiologic® Management of Inferior Vena Cava Filters. Reston, VA: American College of Radiology; 2012:1–4

[10] Kearon C, Akl EA, Ornelas J, et al. Antithrombotic therapy for VTE disease: CHEST guideline and expert panel report. Chest. 2016; 149(2):315–352

[11] Rogers FB, Cipolle MD, Velmahos G, Rozycki G, Luchette FA. Practice management guidelines for the prevention of venous thromboembolism in trauma patients: the EAST practice management guidelines work group. J Trauma. 2002; 53(1): 142–164

[12] Jaff MR, McMurtry MS, Archer SL, et al. American Heart Association Council on Cardiopulmonary, Critical Care, Perioperative and Resuscitation, American Heart Association Council on Peripheral Vascular Disease, American Heart Association Council on Arteriosclerosis, Thrombosis and Vascular Biology. Management of massive and submassive pulmonary embolism, iliofemoral deep vein thrombosis, and chronic thromboembolic pulmonary hypertension: a scientific statement from the American Heart Association. Circulation. 2011; 123 (16):1788–1830

[13] Kinney TB. Inferior vena cava filters. Semin Intervent Radiol. 2006; 23(3):230–239

[14] Geerts WH, Heit JA, Clagett GP, et al. Prevention of venous thromboembolism. Chest. 2001; 119(1) Suppl:132S–175S

[15] Caplin DM, Nikolic B, Kalva SP, Ganguli S, Saad WE, Zuckerman DA, Society of Interventional Radiology Standards of Practice Committee. Quality improvement guidelines for the performance of inferior vena cava filter placement for the prevention of pulmonary embolism. J Vasc Interv Radiol. 2011; 22(11):1499–1506

[16] Deso SE, Idakoji IA, Kuo WT. Evidence-based evaluation of inferior vena cava filter complications based on filter type. Semin Intervent Radiol. 2016; 33(2):93–100

[17] Andreoli JM, Lewandowski RJ, Vogelzang RL, Ryu RK. Comparison of complication rates associated with permanent and retrievable inferior vena cava filters: a review of the MAUDE database. J Vasc Interv Radiol. 2014; 25(8):1181–1185

[18] US Food and Drug Administration (FDA). Inferior vena cava (IVC) filters: initial communication—risk of adverse events with long term use. 2017–2018. 2018. Accessed March 14, 2024 at: https://wayback.archive-it.org/7993/201701121656 20/http://www.fda.gov/Safety/MedWatch/SafetyInformation/ SafetyAlertsforHumanMedicalProducts/ucm221707.htm

[19] Jones TK, Barnes RW, Greenfield LJ. Greenfield vena caval filter: rationale and current indications. Ann Thorac Surg. 1986; 42(6) Suppl:S48–S55

[20] Minocha J, Idakoji I, Riaz A, et al. Improving inferior vena cava filter retrieval rates: impact of a dedicated inferior vena cava filter clinic. J Vasc Interv Radiol. 2010; 21(12):1847–1851

Chapter 6

Retrievable Inferior Vena Cava Filters: Challenges in Device Utilization, Advanced Retrieval Techniques to Optimize Outcomes

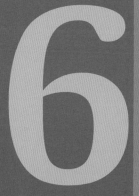

6 Retrievable Inferior Vena Cava Filters: Challenges in Device Utilization, Advanced Retrieval Techniques to Optimize Outcomes

Nicholas Xiao, Karan S. Gulaya, Robert J. Lewandowski, and Kush R. Desai

Keywords: inferior vena cava filter, venous thromboembolism, deep vein thrombosis, pulmonary embolism

6.1 Introduction

Inferior vena cava filters (IVCFs) have become an important tool in the treatment of patients with venous thromboembolic disease (VTE) who have contraindications to, or previous failed treatment with, medical anticoagulation.[1,2] These devices effectively decrease the short-term risk of pulmonary embolism (PE); however, they also increase the risk of thrombotic events such as deep venous thrombosis or caval occlusion.[3,4,5,6] Furthermore, nonthrombotic complications, such as filter penetration into adjacent structures, device fracture, migration and embolism, and even death have also been reported.[5,7,8,9,10,11] As no long-term benefit of IVCF has been proven, retrievable IVCFs (rIVCFs) were developed to offer temporary protection from PE with the intention of filter removal once the device was no longer indicated, thereby avoiding the risk of filter-related adverse events.

The introduction of rIVCFs into clinical practice has resulted in dramatic increases in device utilization.[12,13] Although these devices were designed to be removed when no longer needed, most rIVCFs are left in patients permanently.[14,15] Studies have demonstrated low retrieval rates of these filters, much of which is attributed to poor patient follow-up.[16] As implantation time increases, retrieval can become increasingly difficult; up to 60% of long-dwelling rIVCF become embedded into the caval wall; retrieval of these devices with standard retrieval techniques frequently fails.[15,16,17] Reported retrieval failure rates are as high as 43% in prolonged dwell times.[17] Consequently, patients with rIVCFs are frequently left with a permanent device, often unintentionally.[13,18] Further complicating matters is that prolonged rIVCF implantation times have also been associated with increasing rates of both thrombotic and nonthrombotic, filter-related complications.[3,4,5] These issues are mirrored in a 2014 US Food and Drug Administration (FDA) safety communication, highlighting the importance of device retrieval once it is no longer indicated.[19]

This chapter discusses key clinical issues in the utilization of rIVCFs and will examine advanced techniques used in the retrieval of embedded filters.

6.2 Permanent versus Retrievable IVCFs

Permanent IVCFs (pIVCFs) were the initial device type to enter clinical practice in 1968, followed by the introduction of rIVCFs in 2003. Although both have been cleared by the FDA for permanent implantation, significant differences exist between rIVCF and pIVCF. Retrievable filters are engineered with the intention of removal when no longer indicated, thereby presenting an interesting challenge for device design. The device must not only offer mechanical embolic protection and maintain its position in the inferior vena cava (IVC), but also must be easily and safely manipulable facilitating retrieval. Although studies have shown that rIVCFs are effective in mitigating risks of PE, it has also been shown that they are much more likely to fracture, migrate/embolize, or penetrate into nearby structures as compared to their pIVCF counterparts.[3,8,10,11,20] Literature on rIVCF adverse events have reported complication rates of 9% and that as high as 87% of user-reported events were associated with rIVCF as opposed to 13% with pIVCF.[20,21] Both thrombotic and nonthrombotic events increase directly with implantation time, particularly device fracture and embolization.[18,22,23] As dwell time increases, these filters experience "metal fatigue," as they are deteriorated by additive biomechanical rotational and torsional forces in situ, thereby weakening structural integrity.[22,24] This developing understanding of in situ device behavior, as well as the downstream consequences, has led to renewed clinical and regulatory emphasis on device retrieval when no longer indicated.[25]

6.3 Obstacles to Filter Retrieval

Clinical follow-up of patients with rIVCFs has been poor since their inception, with select studies reporting retrieval rates as low as 8.5%.[26] Placement and retrieval of rIVCF are performed by multiple medical specialties, such as interventional radiology, cardiology, and vascular surgery, significantly complicating monitoring of patients with implanted devices and impeding clinical follow-up for retrieval when filters are no longer indicated. Recent studies revealed that interventional radiologists placed and retrieved the majority of filters (60.4 and 63.5%, respectively).[13] The development of dedicated service lines for patients with rIVCF is critical, with one study reporting an increase in retrieval rates by more than 30% after the establishment of a dedicated IVCF service.[27]

A second major impediment to retrieval of rIVCF is prolonged dwell time. Several studies have identified longer implantation times as a negative predictor for successful retrieval, with one study in 200 patients noting that dwell times over 90 days was significantly associated with retrieval failure and a second study noting an increased likelihood of failure at 6 months.[28,29] These reports have led to the perception by operators and referring physicians that retrieval of rIVCF with prolonged dwell times should not be attempted due to the futility of retrieval, or due to theoretical risks of vascular and perivascular injury during retrieval.[30] However, recent literature utilizing advanced filter retrieval techniques have shown that regardless of dwell time, filter retrieval success can be as high as 97% with low complication rates.[31] In concordance with this finding and with the underlying pathophysiology of filter embedment, filters with longer implantation times required advanced filter retrieval techniques more often for successful device removal.[31,32] Although these advanced techniques are often complex and utilize devices in an off-label manner such as endobronchial forceps or a xenon chloride (XeCl) excimer laser, complication rates remain very low and are not correlated with dwell time.[31] More recently, a single-center study demonstrated that advanced filter retrieval techniques were necessary after 7 months implantation time; knowledge of this time point can be helpful in patient triage to centers with retrieval expertise.[33]

6.4 Filter Types and Removal Techniques

Retrievable filters can be conical, polyhedron, or helical in design. Examples of frequently deployed conical filters are the Denali, G2X/G2, Eclipse, and Meridian (Bard Peripheral Vascular Inc., Tempe, AZ), Celect and Gunther Tulip (Cook Medical Inc., Bloomington, IN), ALN (ALN Implants Chirurgicaux, GHisonaccia, France), and Option/Option Elite (Argon Medical Devices, Plano, TX). The OptEase (Cordis Corp., Miami Lakes, FL) has a nonconical polyhedron structure and the Crux (Volcano Corp., San Diego, CA) has a helical design. Conical filters are engineered with hooks on the cranial end of the device intended to facilitate engagement of the device and are therefore designed to be retrieved via an internal jugular vein access site. The OptEase is designed to be retrieved from a femoral venous access, while the Crux contains hooks on both the caudal and cranial aspects of the filter, allowing retrieval from either the jugular or femoral approach. This section will detail standard and advanced filter retrieval techniques.

6.4.1 Standard Technique

The principle of standard retrieval of rIVCF is to use an endovascular snare device to engage the filter, followed by advancement of a sheath to coaxially collapse the filter and disengage the filter elements from the caval wall. Although many rIVCF manufactures have developed proprietary retrieval kits, in our experience, these are rarely necessary, as rIVCF can be typically retrieved with commonly stocked endovascular sheath snares.

Our standard filter retrieval procedure begins with a pigtail flush catheter which is introduced over a wire caudal to the filter; care must be taken not to entangle the wire within filter. Venography of the IVC is performed to assess for in situ filter thrombus. Coaxial sheaths are then introduced immediately cranial to the filter. A standard endovascular snare is subsequently employed to capture the filter hook. Once the filter is successfully captured and engaged, gentle "equal and opposite" traction/counter-traction is applied using the snare and the sheath, resulting in collapse and explantation of the filter.

6.4.2 Advanced Retrieval Techniques

Standard rIVCF retrieval techniques often fail to successfully remove rIVCF, particularly with extended implantation times.[15,34] Common reasons include filter tilt or encasement of the filter hook by a fibrin cap, both of which limit access to the device by an endovascular snare. Incorporation of filter elements into the caval wall, with or without significant extracaval perforation of filter struts, or filter fracture also significantly complicates retrieval of these devices. Advanced retrieval techniques have been developed to successfully mitigate these obstacles and safely permit device retrieval.

When filters are significantly tilted, standard straight sheaths and snare devices are often not able to successful engage the filter hook. Therefore, a curved inner sheath can be employed to give the operator directional control of the devices and can facilitate snaring of a hook that is greatly deviated from the central axis of the IVC (▶ Fig. 6.1). In our practice, we use a Flexor sheath with Ansel 2 modification (Cook Medical Inc., Bloomington, IN). This technique is most effective if the filter hook is not also embedded into the IVC, and if no fibrin cap is present, inhibiting access to the hook.

One of the most significant challenges in complex filter retrieval arises when the device apex is densely adherent and embedded to the caval wall; in most cases fibrin deposition has obstructed access to the filter apex. Several techniques have been developed as an approach to these complex retrievals. In our practice, we utilize the loop snare and rigid endobronchial forceps.

The loop-snare technique employed at our institution is a modified version of the original description in the literature. Classically, the loop-snare technique is described as follows: a reverse curve catheter is guided through the struts of the filter, and a hydrophilic wire is passed cranially to the device.[30] The free end of the wire is then snared

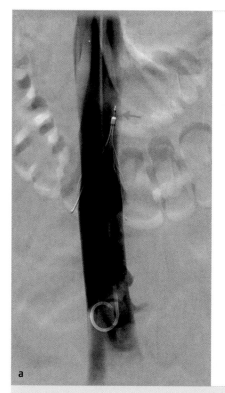
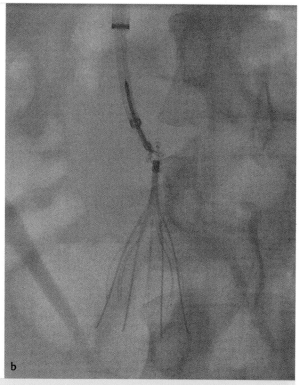

Fig. 6.1 Utilization of a curved sheath for retrieval of nonembedded, tilted filters. **(a)** Filter hook is significantly tilted from the central axis of the cava (green arrow). **(b)** Curved inner sheath provides directionality to the snare device allowing for successful capturing of the displaced filter hook.

and externalized, forming a wire loop. This loop is then utilized to provide counter-traction while the sheath is coaxially collapsed over the filter (▶ Fig. 6.2). This maneuver is not routinely performed at our institution, primarily out of concerns of filter fracture while exerting direct counter-traction forces on the filter components. If the unmodified version of the loop-snare technique is attempted, capturing multiple struts in the formed loop may help reduce fracture events by avoiding the application of excessive force to a single strut. In our modified technique, the fibrin cap is the target of the loop snare instead of the device itself. A reverse curve catheter is used to engage the fibrin cap at the filter apex, and then a hydrophilic wire is advanced cranially and snared forming a wire loop through the fibrin cap (▶ Fig. 6.3).[35] The sheath is then advanced coaxially over the wire loop—this frequently results either in direct collapse and capture of the filter or in disruption and removal of the fibrin cap. If the latter occurs, a standard technique can then be used for trivial retrieval.

Rigid forceps are a malleable instrument and can be shaped with curvature to access tilted and embedded filters. Many different types of forceps are commercially available; the best described are rigid endobronchial forceps (model 4162, Lymol

Medical, Woburn, MA). This device allows for the operator to dissect fibrinous tissue from the filter apex, therefore freeing and exposing the filter hook.[36,37] Once the fibrin encasing the apex has been sufficiently dissected and removed, the filter hook can be easily captured with the forceps and the sheath can be advanced coaxially to collapse and remove the filter (▶ Fig. 6.4). However, care must be taken as tearing of the IVC can occur if the operator engages the caval wall instead of fibrin tissue with the forceps. Furthermore, exaggerated forceps curvature can cause caval distention and great discomfort to the patient. In many cases, when forceps use is predicted during preprocedural planning, patients are scheduled with deep sedation or general anesthesia by coordinating with anesthesiology.

The previously discussed techniques facilitate access to the filter hook, thereby allowing for retrieval. However, in some cases, after successfully capturing the hook, the IVCF cannot be collapsed by the sheath despite the application of very large forces. This frequently is the result of incorporation of the filter struts into the caval wall. When we encounter this problem, we utilize a laser sheath to perform photothermal ablation of fibrinous tissue densely adhering the filter struts into the IVC.[32,38] The CVX-300 XeCl excimer laser system utilizes

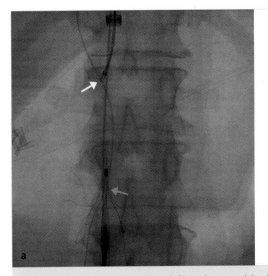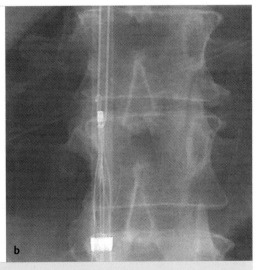

Fig. 6.2 Loop-wire technique through filter elements. **(a)** A hydrophilic wire is passed through a reverse curve catheter and snared (white arrow). Note that the wire is looped through the filter struts and not through the filter hook (green arrow). **(b)** Tension is exerted through the loop-wire and the sheath is coaxially advanced over the filter apex, successfully collapsing the filter.

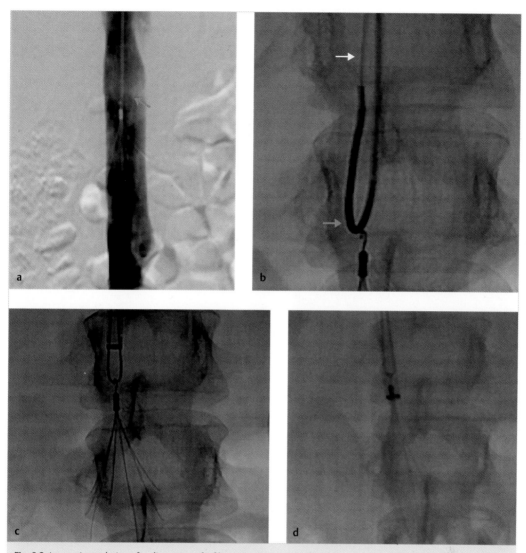

Fig. 6.3 Loop-wire technique for disruption of a fibrin cap. **(a)** Digital subtraction cavogram suggests apical formation of a fibrin cap inhibiting access to the hook of the filter (green arrow). **(b)** Reverse curve catheter engaging the fibrin cap (green arrow). Hydrophilic wire is advanced cranially and captured with snare device, forming the loop-wire (white arrow). **(c)** Loop wire successfully engaged on fibrin cap. The struts of the filter have not been engaged by the wire. **(d)** Utilizing tension and counter-tension forces with the loop wire, the sheath is advanced coaxially over the filter, successfully capturing the device.

12-, 14-, and 16-Fr sheaths (GlideLight, Philips Spectranetics, Colorado Springs, CO), which are introduced via a larger outer sheath. The system is advanced over the filter, until the point of maximal resistance is reached, localizing areas of caval incorporation impeding filter explantation. The laser is then sequentially activated to ablate the encasing tissue. This eventually allows for complete advancement of the sheath and filter collapse and removal (▶ Fig. 6.5). Engagement and control of the filter apex or hook is a prerequisite to employ photothermal ablation, as counter-traction must be applied to collapse the filter. Therefore, it is common that multiple advanced techniques must be used in

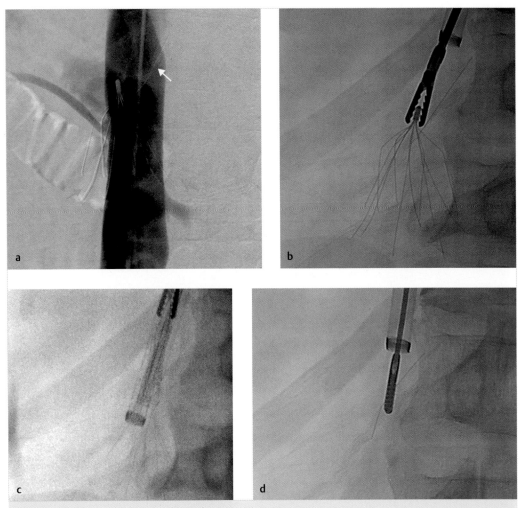

Fig. 6.4 Utilization of rigid endobronchial forceps. **(a)** Digital subtraction cavogram demonstrates a tilted filter with multiple penetrated struts (green arrows) and with device fracture/disfigurement (white arrow). **(b)** Rigid forceps are used to capture the filter apex. **(c)** The filter is successfully collapsed in the sheath and subsequently retrieved. **(d)** A remaining fractured strut is captured and retrieved using the forceps.

conjunction when filters have a fibrin cap inhibiting access to the apex, while also complicated by struts embedded in the IVC.

6.5 Conclusion

rIVCFs are an important and effective tool in protection of patients with contraindications to medical anticoagulation from PE. However, diligent clinical follow-up and monitoring of these patients with implanted filters is critical, as both thrombotic and nonthrombotic complications are associated with these devices and occur at higher rates with increasing dwell times. Advanced filter retrieval techniques allow for safe and successful removal of these filters regardless of their implantation time, and retrieval should be attempted promptly in all patients when the rIVCF is no longer indicated.

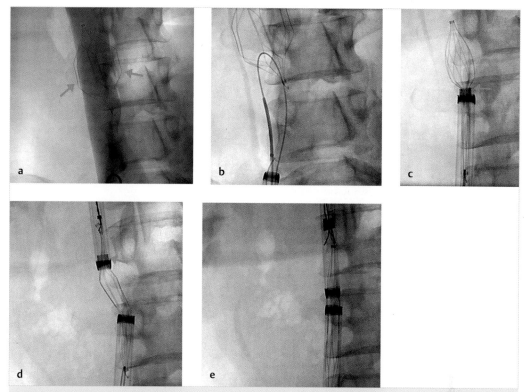

Fig. 6.5 Excimer laser sheath–assisted filter retrieval. **(a)** Digital subtraction cavogram demonstrates incorporation (green arrows) of filter elements into the caval wall. **(b)** A loop-wire technique is used to capture the filter from below. **(c)** The laser sheath (green arrow) is sequentially activated and advanced coaxially, ablating the encasing fibrous tissue at the caudal end. **(d)** Filter elements at the cranial end remain embedded; following successful engagement of the cranial end of the filter, the laser sheath (green arrow) is introduced from the jugular access and activated from above. **(e)** Ablation of fibrous tissues liberates the struts from the caval wall and allows for complete collapse of the filter.

References

[1] Duszak R, Jr, Parker L, Levin DC, Rao VM. Placement and removal of inferior vena cava filters: national trends in the medicare population. J Am Coll Radiol. 2011; 8(7):483–489

[2] Kearon C, Akl EA, Ornelas J, et al. Antithrombotic therapy for VTE disease: CHEST guideline and expert panel report. Chest. 2016; 149(2):315–352

[3] Group PS, PREPIC Study Group. Eight-year follow-up of patients with permanent vena cava filters in the prevention of pulmonary embolism: the PREPIC (Prevention du Risque d'Embolie Pulmonaire par Interruption Cave) randomized study. Circulation. 2005; 112(3):416–422

[4] Decousus H, Leizorovicz A, Parent F, et al. A clinical trial of vena caval filters in the prevention of pulmonary embolism in patients with proximal deep-vein thrombosis. Prévention du Risque d'Embolie Pulmonaire par Interruption Cave Study Group. N Engl J Med. 1998; 338(7):409–415

[5] McLoney ED, Krishnasamy VP, Castle JC, Yang X, Guy G. Complications of Celect, Günther tulip, and Greenfield inferior vena cava filters on CT follow-up: a single-institution experience. J Vasc Interv Radiol. 2013; 24(11):1723–1729

[6] Millward SF, Oliva VL, Bell SD, et al. Günther Tulip Retrievable Vena Cava Filter: results from the Registry of the Canadian Interventional Radiology Association. J Vasc Interv Radiol. 2001; 12(9):1053–1058

[7] Tam MD, Spain J, Lieber M, Geisinger M, Sands MJ, Wang W. Fracture and distant migration of the Bard Recovery filter: a retrospective review of 363 implantations for potentially life-threatening complications. J Vasc Interv Radiol. 2012; 23(2): 199–205.e1

[8] Durack JC, Westphalen AC, Kekulawela S, et al. Perforation of the IVC: rule rather than exception after longer indwelling times for the Günther Tulip and Celect retrievable filters. Cardiovasc Intervent Radiol. 2012; 35(2):299–308

[9] Ford ME, Lippert JA, McGraw JK. Symptomatic filter penetration presenting as pancreatitis. J Vasc Interv Radiol. 2010; 21 (4):574–576

[10] Malgor RD, Labropoulos N. A systematic review of symptomatic duodenal perforation by inferior vena cava filters. J Vasc Surg. 2012; 55(3):856–861.e3

[11] Putterman D, Niman D, Cohen G. Aortic pseudoaneurysm after penetration by a Simon nitinol inferior vena cava filter. J Vasc Interv Radiol. 2005; 16(4):535–538

[12] Smouse B, Johar A. Is market growth of vena cava filters justified? Endovascular Today. 2010(February):74–77

[13] Ahmed O, Wadhwa V, Patel K, Patel MV, Turba UC, Arslan B. Rising retrieval rates of inferior vena cava filters in the United States: insights from the 2012 to 2016 summary Medicare claims data. J Am Coll Radiol. 2018; 15(11):1553–1557

[14] Helling TS, Kaswan S, Miller SL, Tretter JF. Practice patterns in the use of retrievable inferior vena cava filters in a trauma population: a single-center experience. J Trauma. 2009; 67 (6):1293–1296

[15] Ray CE, Jr, Mitchell E, Zipser S, Kao EY, Brown CF, Moneta GL. Outcomes with retrievable inferior vena cava filters: a multi-center study. J Vasc Interv Radiol. 2006; 17(10):1595–1604

[16] Gaspard SF, Gaspard DJ. Retrievable inferior vena cava filters are rarely removed. Am Surg. 2009; 75(5):426–428

[17] Marquess JS, Burke CT, Beecham AH, et al. Factors associated with failed retrieval of the Günther Tulip inferior vena cava filter. J Vasc Interv Radiol. 2008; 19(9):1321–1327

[18] Kuo WT, Robertson SW, Odegaard JI, Hofmann LV. Complex retrieval of fractured, embedded, and penetrating inferior vena cava filters: a prospective study with histologic and electron microscopic analysis. J Vasc Interv Radiol. 2013; 24 (5):622–630.e1, quiz 631

[19] Administration USFDA. Removing Retrievable Inferior Vena Cava Filters: FDA Safety Communication. https://www.fdagov/ MedicalDevices/Safety/AlertsandNotices/ucm396377htm. 2014

[20] Andreoli JM, Lewandowski RJ, Vogelzang RL, Ryu RK. Comparison of complication rates associated with permanent and retrievable inferior vena cava filters: a review of the MAUDE database. J Vasc Interv Radiol. 2014; 25(8):1181–1185

[21] Desai TR, Morcos OC, Lind BB, et al. Complications of indwelling retrievable versus permanent inferior vena cava filters. J Vasc Surg Venous Lymphat Disord. 2014; 2(2):166–173

[22] Laborda A, Sierre S, Malvè M, et al. Influence of breathing movements and Valsalva maneuver on vena caval dynamics. World J Radiol. 2014; 6(10):833–839

[23] Nicholson W, Nicholson WJ, Tolerico P, et al. Prevalence of fracture and fragment embolization of Bard retrievable vena cava filters and clinical implications including cardiac perforation and tamponade. Arch Intern Med. 2010; 170(20): 1827–1831

[24] Kuo WT, Robertson SW. Bard Denali inferior vena cava filter fracture and embolization resulting in cardiac tamponade: a device failure analysis. J Vasc Interv Radiol. 2015; 26(1): 111–115.e1

[25] Administration USFaD. Removing Retrievable Inferior Vena Cava Filters: Initial Communication. http://wwwfdagov/ MedicalDevices/Safety/AlertsandNotices/ucm221676htm

[26] Sarosiek S, Crowther M, Sloan JM. Indications, complications, and management of inferior vena cava filters: the experience in 952 patients at an academic hospital with a level I trauma center. JAMA Intern Med. 2013; 173(7):513–517

[27] Minocha J, Idakoji I, Riaz A, et al. Improving inferior vena cava filter retrieval rates: impact of a dedicated inferior vena cava filter clinic. J Vasc Interv Radiol. 2010; 21(12): 1847–1851

[28] Geisbüsch P, Benenati JF, Peña CS, et al. Retrievable inferior vena cava filters: factors that affect retrieval success. Cardiovasc Intervent Radiol. 2012; 35(5):1059–1065

[29] Rosenthal D, Wellons ED, Hancock SM, Burkett AB. Retrievability of the Günther Tulip vena cava filter after dwell times longer than 180 days in patients with multiple trauma. J Endovasc Ther. 2007; 14(3):406–410

[30] Rubenstein L, Chun AK, Chew M, Binkert CA. Loop-snare technique for difficult inferior vena cava filter retrievals. J Vasc Interv Radiol. 2007; 18(10):1315–1318

[31] Desai KR, Lewandowski RJ, Salem R, et al. Retrieval of inferior vena cava filters with prolonged dwell time: a single-center experience in 648 retrieval procedures. JAMA Intern Med. 2015; 175(9):1572–1574

[32] Kuo WT, Cupp JS. The excimer laser sheath technique for embedded inferior vena cava filter removal. J Vasc Interv Radiol. 2010; 21(12):1896–1899

[33] Desai KR, Laws JL, Salem R, et al. Defining prolonged dwell time: when are advanced inferior vena cava filter retrieval techniques necessary? An analysis in 762 procedures. Circ Cardiovasc Interv. 2017; 10(6):e003957

[34] Angel LF, Tapson V, Galgon RE, Restrepo MI, Kaufman J. Systematic review of the use of retrievable inferior vena cava filters. J Vasc Interv Radiol. 2011; 22(11):1522–1530.e3

[35] Esparaz AM, Ryu RK, Gupta R, Resnick SA, Salem R, Lewandowski RJ. Fibrin cap disruption: an adjunctive technique for inferior vena cava filter retrieval. J Vasc Interv Radiol. 2012; 23(9):1233–1235

[36] Stavropoulos SW, Dixon RG, Burke CT, et al. Embedded inferior vena cava filter removal: use of endobronchial forceps. J Vasc Interv Radiol. 2008; 19(9):1297–1301

[37] Stavropoulos SW, Ge BH, Mondschein JI, Shlansky-Goldberg RD, Sudheendra D, Trerotola SO. Retrieval of tip-embedded inferior vena cava filters by using the endobronchial forceps technique: experience at a single institution. Radiology. 2015; 275(3):900–907

[38] Kuo WT, Odegaard JI, Rosenberg JK, Hofmann LV. Laser-assisted removal of embedded vena cava filters: a 5-year first-in-human study. Chest. 2017; 151(2):417–424

Chapter 7

Inferior Vena Caval and Right Atrial Thrombus

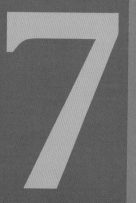

7 Inferior Vena Caval and Right Atrial Thrombus

Scott Resnick

Keywords: clot in transit, right atrial thrombus

7.1 Introduction

Inferior vena cava (IVC) thrombosis and right atrial (RA) thrombosis are both less prevalent, high morbidity and mortality subsets of deep venous thrombosis. Due to the variability in presentation of IVC thrombosis, the exact annual prevalence of the disease remains elusive. However, IVC thrombosis is present in approximately 2.6 to 4.0% of patients with lower extremity deep vein thrombosis (DVT).[1] The mortality rate from IVC thrombosis is twice as high as that of DVT confined to the lower extremities.[2] If left untreated, patients with IVC thrombosis are at high risk for significant morbidities, such as post-thrombotic syndrome in up to 90%, disabling venous claudication in 45%, pulmonary embolism (PE) in 30%, and venous ulceration in 15%.[3,4] One of the most common causes of IVC thrombosis is congenital caval abnormalities that are estimated to be prevalent in as high as 60 to 80% patients with caval thrombus.[1] In a congenitally normal IVC, thrombosis is rare and is usually caused by either acquired pathology such as malignancy, hematological abnormalities, or mechanical factors causing turbulent flow. Implanted IVC filters have become a major predisposing factor for acquired IVC thrombosis with published rates of caval thrombosis after filter implantation ranging from 2 to 30%.[5,6]

Compared to the IVC thrombosis, RA thrombosis is a much less studied phenomenon with a complex multifactorial pathophysiology. Similar to the IVC, RA clot formation is a product of mechanical, hematological, and intrinsic factors. According to Casazza et al, the prevalence of RA thrombosis is unclear and identification rates are dependent upon the timing of atrial imaging, with a greater likelihood for RA thrombus identification when performed earlier in the patients' treatment course.[7] Thrombi originating in the RA are also more common in patients with atrial flow disturbance such as atrial fibrillation or implanted intracardiac devices, such as pacemaker leads or indwelling catheters. According to the International Cooperative Pulmonary Embolism Registry (ICOPER) study, in patients with right heart thrombosis, the prevalence of atrial fibrillation is 12%.[8] In patients with central venous catheters, the incidence of right heart thrombus has been shown to be as high as 12.5%.[9] RA thrombi are also seen in patients with mechanical and prosthetic valves.

7.2 Etiologies

Venous thromboembolism (VTE) etiologies can be broadly divided into congenital versus acquired. The causes of congenital thromboembolism include congenital vessel defect/malformation and coagulopathies, while acquired thromboembolism is comprised of abdominal/chest pathology and acquired coagulopathy. Congenital coagulopathies may remain asymptomatic in individuals for many years due to the mechanisms involved in angiogenesis and collateral flow. On the other hand, acquired thrombosis can be attributed to a wide range of prothrombotic pathologic factors. These predisposing factors include acquired coagulopathies (malignancy, oral contraceptive use, pregnancy, hormonal replacement therapy, and nephrotic syndrome among others) as well as new-onset pathology in the abdomen (masses, trauma, Budd-Chiari, May–Thurner, and IVC filters) or chest (masses, trauma, implanted devices, vegetations, and valvular lesions).

It is important to note that an overlap exists between congenital and acquired etiologies causing increased propensity for developing VTEs. Virchow broadly described three predisposing factors for thrombosis, resulting in the eponymous triad, namely, endothelial injury, hypercoagulable state, and turbulence/stasis. Pathologies that affect each of these factors can be assumed to increase the overall likelihood of thrombosis, and in our case IVC/RA thrombosis specifically. Many of the predisposing factors are well known to us. For example, known factors that cause endothelial damage include trauma, surgery, or presence of an intravascular device. Common factors that cause turbulence/stasis include: prolonged immobilization, compressive masses, intravenous devices, and pregnancy. Finally, factors that cause hypercoagulable state have already been mentioned.

7.2.1 Congenital IVC Anomalies

Most congenital venous anomalies remain asymptomatic for years due to the development of collateral circulation blood flow. They are often discovered as incidental findings during routine imaging. However, any insult to the collateral vessels or the remaining patent channel can lead to acute venous thrombosis. It is estimated that the prevalence of the IVC anomalies in the general population is around 0.3 to 0.6%, with the lifetime IVC thrombosis risk of 60 to 80%.[10,11] There seems to be a high association between congenital IVC anomalies and thrombophilia in early-onset IVC thrombosis, suggesting that the presence of a hypercoagulable state might tip the fragile balance of collateral circulation in patients with congenital IVC anomalies toward thrombosis.[12]

In contradistinction to IVC thrombosis which usually results from in situ caval clot development or direct extension of clot from the iliac veins, RA thrombi are almost always multifactorial in origin, often involving a combination of mechanical, hematological, and intrinsic factors. Felner et al found that although RA thromboembolism can result from in situ development due to RA stasis from atrial fibrillation or a decreased cardiac output from congestive heart failure, it is more common secondary to an insult from a foreign body or an embolization from a remote site.[13] The most common pathway for RA thrombosis is remote clot formation with subsequent migration to the right atrium, commonly known as "thrombus in transit." Once the clot is in the right atrium it may adhere and grow larger secondary to flow perturbation or it may embolize to the pulmonary vasculature. The exact prevalence of RA thrombosis remains elusive. According to Casazza et al, in the presence of massive PE, the prevalence of RA thrombosis depends on the timing of the echocardiography performed, since the earlier the sonography is performed the more likely RA thrombi will be found.[7] The presumption being that at delayed imaging the clot in transit may have exited the atrium and moved into the pulmonary circulation.

7.2.2 Congenital Coagulopathies

There are a myriad of genetic determinants for VTE. These genetic variants can be broadly grouped into those that causes either deficiency of antithrombotic factors or excess of prothrombotic factors, leading to a hypercoagulable state that makes formation of a thrombus (IVC and RA included) more likely. Of the various thrombophilias, Factor V Leiden is the most common cause of VTE. This coagulopathy occurs in 5 to 15% of the population and is transmitted in an autosomal dominant fashion.[14] The risk of VTE is 30- to 140-fold with the homozygous mutation and 3- to 6-fold with the heterozygous mutation.[15] The second most common inherited coagulopathy is mutation in prothrombin gene which is also transmitted in an autosomal dominant fashion. This mutation occurs approximately 1.1 to 3% in the population and is associated with a threefold increased risk of VTE.[16]

Other, less common but still important, mutations included antithrombin III (ATIII) deficiency and protein C and S deficiencies. Antithrombin III is a serine protease inhibitor that acts as a natural anticoagulant, inactivating multiple coagulation factors, while proteins C and S act on the platelet surface to inactivate both procoagulation factors Va and VIIIa. The deficiency in either protein C or S therefore manifests into a coagulopathic state. Mutations in production of either protein present with 2 to 5% incidence of VTE.[17] It is important to note that antithrombin or protein C and S deficiencies can also be acquired through decreased protein production in liver failure or through protein loss via nephrotic syndrome.

Additionally, high incidence of VTE has been reported in sickle cell disease and hyperhomocysteinemia. There is evidence that venous thrombosis is a common feature of sickle cell disease especially during sickling crisis showing depletion of anticoagulant proteins and increase in coagulation markers. Increased homocysteine levels have been shown to be associated with venous and arterial thrombosis. Inherited hyperhomocysteinemia occurs from mutations within the homocysteine production and metabolism pathways. The pathophysiology of prothrombotic state from hyperhomocysteinemia remains unclear but it has been speculated that it involves impaired endothelium-dependent regulation of blood flow causing increase in inflammatory mediators.[18]

7.2.3 Acquired Coagulopathies

In addition to genetic causes of hypercoagulable states, acquired thrombophilias also increase the risk of thrombus formation, IVC and RA included. The more common acquired coagulopathies are heparin-induced thrombocytopenia (HIT), thrombotic thrombocytopenic purpura, and antiphospholipid syndrome (APS), all of which involve endogenous antibody production that promotes a procoagulation state. Common acquired coagulopathies such as malignancy, pregnancy, obesity, and immobilization are assumed to be universally well understood and will not be discussed in detail. Other acquired hypercoagulable conditions, such as cryoglobulinemia and cryofibrinogenemia, are much less common and will also not be discussed.

HIT is a commonly encountered acquired thrombophilia and results from an immunological reaction to heparin resulting in antibody formation causing a paradoxical heparin-induced prothrombotic state, rather than the expected anticoagulation effect. HIT occurs due to production of heparin/platelet-dependent antibodies following heparin administration. The clinical picture is that of the diminishing platelet count with intravascular arterial and venous thrombosis following heparin administration. The prevalence of HIT has been estimated to be around 1 to 5% in patients receiving heparin.[19] On the other hand, thrombotic-thrombocytopenia purpura (TTP) can manifest as either an inherited or acquired condition. The inherited form involves a defect in the von Willebrand Factor (vWF) cleaving protein, ADAMTS13, resulting in accumulation of vWF multimers within the endothelium causing thrombocytopenia, microangiopathic hemolytic anemia, and widespread thrombosis. Acquired TTP involves production of anti-ADAMTS13 antibodies and has been associated with connective tissue disease, human immunodeficiency virus (HIV), and cytomegalovirus (CMV) infections, as well as with certain medications.

Lastly, APS is a hypercoagulable state characterized by prothrombosis due to antibodies against phospholipid-binding proteins. These antiphospholipid antibodies include: lupus anticoagulant, anticardiolipin antibody, and anti-beta-2-glycoprotein antibody. APS can occur either without an obvious trigger or it can be induced by autoimmunity, medications, infection, and malignancy. Multiple etiologic mechanisms have been suggested and involve activation of platelets, endothelial cells, and proinflammatory state.

7.2.4 Medical Devices

Any implanted intravenous medical device has a potential to cause venous thrombosis. These devices, including peripheral and central intravenous catheters, tunneled and nontunneled central catheters, ports and rhythm maintenance devices, IVC filters, and others can potentially cause local endothelial injury resulting in local thrombus formation or can act as a nidus for infection with a secondary increased thrombotic rate. There is a wide variation in the incidence of vein thrombosis depending on the catheter type and catheter location. The study by Forauer and Theoharis showed that short-term catheter placement can result in local endothelial injury, while a long-term placement results in vein wall thickening and fibrin bridge formation from the adjacent vein to the catheter creating a turbulent flow and facilitating further fibrin deposition and clot formation.[20]

The use of central venous catheters (CVCs) in clinical practice has been on the rise. These CVCs have an estimated 27 to 67% incidence of asymptomatic catheter-associated DVT.[21,22] A certain portion of these CVC-associated thrombus patients will also have RA clot. An autopsy study on 141 patients with CVCs showed the incidence of right heart mural thrombi to be 29%.[23] However, in a study done by Gilon et al, 55 patients showed the associated incidence of right heart thromboembolism to be 12.5%. Gilon et al pointed out that the increased incidence of atrial thrombosis was associated with several mechanical factors including catheter tip placement in the right atrium as opposed to the SVC and acquired prothrombotic states (malignancy, infection, and structural abnormalities).[9] It is without a doubt that many patients requiring CVC placement have underlying conditions that coincidentally places them in the procoagulable state. Further, it has been shown that larger diameters of catheters may play a role in thrombosis since larger catheter diameter can result in increased turbulent flow within the vessel and larger surface area for thrombi adhesion (▶ Fig. 7.1).

7.2.5 IVC Filtration

IVC filters (IVCFs) are currently one of the major predisposing factors causing caval thrombosis in the United States.[2] IVC device utilization has been on the rise, with a steep spike in use following the advent of retrievable filters. It is estimated that approximately 259,000 IVCFs were placed in 2012 and the numbers have been increasing[24] until recently when widespread awareness of IVCF

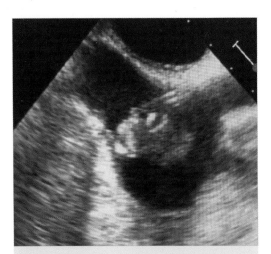

Fig. 7.1 Transesophageal echocardiography (TEE) image of right atrial thrombus associated with the indwelling dialysis catheter.

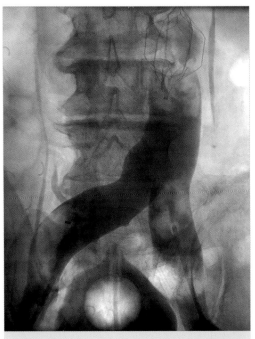

Fig. 7.2 Venogram showing thrombotic caval occlusion and nonocclusive bilateral iliac vein clot with Trapease filter in place.

litigation has led to a declining use curve. The increased device utilization is attributed to the retrievable filters being placed for extended indications, such as prophylaxis in trauma or preoperative patients undergoing orthopedic, neurosurgical, and bariatric procedures.[25] The main goal behind IVCF placement is to trap the thrombi in transit to the lungs. However, IVCFs can potentially cause IVC obstruction through new local thrombus formation in the periphery of the device or through extension of the trapped embolus. Published rates in IVC thrombosis after IVCF placement vary widely from as little as 2% to as high as 30%. The variability is further increased when comparing permanent and retrievable filters, as well as the various specific filter configurations.[5,6] In a meta-analysis performed by Deso et al to identify device-specific complications on Food and Drug Administration (FDA)-approved filters used during 1980 to 2014, the permanent filters with cylindrical component (Vena Tech LGM, Trapease, B Braun Interventional Systems, Bethlehem, Pennsylvania) and umbrella elements (Simon Nitinol, Bard Peripheral Vascular, Tempe, Arizona) were associated with highest rates of caval thrombosis.[26] Of the temporary filters, the Optease retrievable filter was associated with highest degree of caval thrombosis. In fact, Corriere et al have described Trapese and Optease filters having a reported IVC occlusion rates as high as 28.6%.[27] Thrombosis of some of these filters could be potentially due to poor mechanical design

that creates a turbulent flow or acts a nidus for thrombi adhesion. However, a component of the high caval thrombosis rates seen with implanted IVCFs may be explained by the underlying comorbid prothrombotic conditions present in patients indicated for IVC filtration (▶ Fig. 7.2).

7.2.6 Intracardiac Devices

Long-term placement of any intracardiac devices such rhythm maintenance devices and infusion catheters can lead to bacterial and sterile atrial vegetation formation due to local injury or device thrombus accumulation. Such vegetation can occur on either the atrial wall or the adjacent atrial valve. In rare instances the thrombotic accumulations can grow to become quite large and pose a risk of embolization. Contrary to the rates seen with other implanted intracardiac devices, thrombosis/ vegetation formation associated with prosthetic, porcine, or bovine valves is quite low with the incidence reported to be between 0.1 and 5.7% per patient-year.[28] Current guidelines for treatment of endocarditis recommend immediate

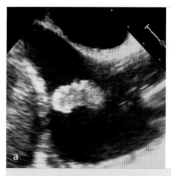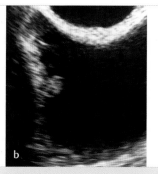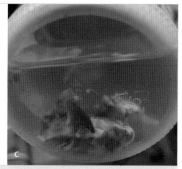

Fig. 7.3 (a) Transesophageal echocardiography (TEE) image of right atrial thrombus. **(b)** TEE image of right atrium following near-total thrombus extraction with AngioVac. **(c)** Specimen of removed right atrial material (chronic thrombus on pathologic evaluation).

early intervention.[29] However, primary surgical atrial intervention can lead to significant perioperative morbidity and mortality and therefore interest in percutaneous extraction is increasing (▶ Fig. 7.3).

7.3 Diagnosis

Patients with IVC thrombosis often present with signs and symptoms similar to uncomplicated lower extremity DVT characterized by leg heaviness, pain, and swelling. Some patients with caval thrombosis may also have nonspecific back and abdominal pain, or other findings not seen with simple extremity DVT, such as scrotal swelling. When chronic, IVC occlusion will often lead to the development of visible anterior body wall collaterals which can aid in diagnosis. Given the myriad of collateral pathways bridging IVC stenosis or occlusion at various levels, those individuals with caval thrombosis may have minimal symptoms. Thus, the diagnosis is often not made until acute caval clot migrates to the pulmonary system or until cross-sectional imaging is obtained.

7.3.1 Diagnostic Imaging—IVC

Diagnosis of IVC thrombosis can be challenging at times due to the nonspecific presentation. In patients with leg DVT in whom additional signs or symptoms suggestive of possible iliocaval thrombosis are present, there should be a low threshold for abdominopelvic imaging as the diagnosis cannot be consistently made without cross-sectional imaging and thrombus visualization. Although

some authors believe a dedicated IVC ultrasound should be the screening modality of choice,[1] others feel strongly that contrast-enhanced computed tomography (CT) should be preferred. The unique combination of operator- and patient-independent image quality, high image resolution, and the added ability to readily identify additional causative or contributory factors such as malignancy are unparalleled benefits of CT imaging. In contrast, the operator-dependent nature of the modality and patient-specific technical challenges presented by such factors as bowel gas or body habitus make caval ultrasound less consistently diagnostic. Kandpal et al concur that CT and MR represent the most sensitive modalities in caval thrombosis testing.[30] Some authors have suggested that the most consistent caval contrast opacification can be achieved with lower extremity contrast injection.[31] Although this technique offers the obvious benefit of contrast-enhanced evaluation of one or both lower extremities, the nonstandard nature of foot IV access in CT scanner workflow makes routine use of this method unlikely.

Further, MR venography has been suggested as the technique of choice for caval imaging when associated malignancy is considered. That said, routine MRI of the abdomen for caval evaluation is limited compared to CT by metallic artifact from implanted devices such as IVCFs. In the patients with such implanted devices within or near the area in question, CT should be the modality of choice.

7.3.2 Diagnostic Imaging RA

RA thrombi are most commonly diagnosed by transesophageal echocardiography (TEE) in patients with suspected or proven PE[32] or at times are identified incidentally in patients undergoing cardiac evaluation. The most common RA thrombus location site is at the junction of the superior vena cava and right atrium.[33] The echocardiographic appearance of acute thromboemboli is distinct from that of mural thrombi, which tend to be more chronic. Such longer duration thrombus shows less motion during the cardiac cycle, although a spectrum of appearance certainly exists, as acutely embolized lower extremity or iliocaval thrombus can become adherent to the atrial wall and remain in situ chronically. Atrial filling defects are on occasion identified incidentally on chest CT imaging. These findings are typically indistinct secondary to cardiac motion, even in those cases where cardiac gating techniques are utilized, and such findings should be followed up by more detailed imaging via TEE.

7.4 Medical Management

Unless contraindicated, anticoagulation should be initiated at the time of diagnosis to prevent thrombus progression. Until recently, anticoagulation with intravenous heparin followed by oral warfarin was the mainstay of VTE treatment. As per the American College of Chest Physicians 2016 guidelines, anticoagulation with non-vitamin K oral anticoagulants (novel oral anticoagulants [NOACs]) are now preferred over warfarin and can be started immediately upon diagnosis without a heparin bridge.[34] This recommended therapy change away from warfarin is due to the numerous food–drug interactions of the drug and narrow therapeutic window that requires frequent blood sampling for international normalized ratio (INR) titration. NOACs include: oral direct factor Xa inhibitors such as rivaroxaban and apixaban as well as oral direct thrombin inhibitors such as dabigatran. Additional nonwarfarin alternative anticoagulants are the indirect factor Xa inhibitors, such as subcutaneous fondaparinux, as well as intravenous direct thrombin inhibitors such as argatroban and bivalirudin. Caution should be exercised with prolonged dabigatran use, since increased risk of acute coronary syndromes has been reported.[35] The preferred anticoagulation therapy for pregnant patients or those with active malignancy is subcutaneous low molecular weight heparin.[34]

7.5 Interventional Management

7.5.1 Acute IVC Thrombosis

Catheter-Directed Thrombolysis

Catheter-directed thrombolysis (CDT) is a percutaneous procedure that seeks to dissolve thrombus by injecting a thrombolytic agent directly into the clot through a catheter. CDT is a modality of choice for dissolving an acute clot and may be used in combination with other thrombolytic methods. When compared to high-dose, nonselective systemic intravenous infusions of thrombolytic agents, CDT has shown to decrease lysis time and reduce the risk of bleeding complications by directly delivering high concentrations of low-dose thrombolytic agents to the target,[36] thereby decreasing the amount of thrombolytic agent use and decreasing systemic bleeding complications. Although CDT provides effective treatment for IVC thrombosis, its use also comes with certain risks and disadvantages. Given that bleeding is the most common complication of lytic infusion, patients who are at significant risk for bleeding (postoperative or trauma patients, those with existing intestinal ulceration or inflammation, and those with known intracranial lesions as well as other) should not undergo routine CDT. Disadvantages include the potential need for lengthy infusion times, usually with multiple interval interventions, potential patient discomfort, need for meticulous monitoring for bleeding complications, and longer intensive care stay.[36] Therefore, it is important to tailor therapy toward the individual patient when considering the use of CDT.

In treating patients with CDT, it is important to consider the thrombolytic options available. All thrombolytics act through the plasminogen–plasmin pathway by directly converting plasminogen to plasmin thereby initiating fibrinolysis. Plasmin acts to enzymatically cleave fibrin and break apart the structure and integrity of the thrombus. In choosing a thrombolytic agent for CDT, the options available include alteplase (r-tPA), reteplase (RPA), and tenecteplase (TNK).

The most commonly used agent is alteplase, a recombinant human tPA. Alteplase is often used as the thrombolytic agent of choice for CDT and has been used effectively in the treatment of extensive IVC thrombosis, even in neonates.[37] Reteplase is also a recombinant human plasminogen activator, and its efficacy is equal to tPA but at much higher doses, requiring approximately three times the molar concentration for optimal effect.[38] The use of reteplase in CDT of IVC thrombosis in humans has not been well explored in the literature. Tenecteplase is another recombinant tissue plasminogen activator. When compared to tPA and reteplase, tenecteplase has higher fibrin specificity and is more resistant to inhibition by plasminogen activator inhibitor-1. Preliminary evidence suggests tenecteplase is safe and effective for use in CDT therapy; however, its potential benefits/risks need to be further explored.[39]

Mechanical/Pharmacological Thrombectomy

Due to the risk of hemorrhagic complications during CDT, percutaneous mechanical thrombectomy (PMT) devices have emerged as an advantageous option for the treatment of acute DVT. The various PMT devices perform their function by macerating the thrombus either by adding low-energy, high-frequency ultrasound waves to enhance thrombolysis (EKOS, Bothell, Washington) or via pulsatile saline jets (AngioJet, Possis Medical, Minneapolis, Minnesota).[1] Additionally, there are systems that are designed for whole thrombus removal through suction, such as, AngioVac (Angiodynamics Inc., Latham, New York) (▶ Fig. 7.4). Rotational devices such as the Cleaner (Argon Medical Devices

Inc., Plano Texas) or the Arrow-Trerotola system (Teleflex Inc., Wayne, Pennsylvania) offer a theoretical benefit of IVC clot fragmentation and subsequent improved extraction ability, but this must be balanced against dangers of thrombus fragment distal embolization with PE. Of course, thrombectomy devices may be used in isolation, in combination, or as an adjunct to thrombolytics, as the situation demands.

Cleaner

The Cleaner rotational thrombectomy system (Argon Medical Devices Inc.) is used for PMT and is indicated for mechanical declotting of native vessel dialysis fistula and synthetic dialysis access grafts and in the peripheral vasculature. It effectively macerates intralumenal and wall-adherent thrombus and has an atraumatic S-wave wire design. Studies suggest that the Cleaner rotational thrombectomy system appears to be safe and effective in the treatment of DVT, but further studies are needed to determine long-term outcomes.[40,41,42] Overall, the use of the Cleaner in caval thrombectomy has not been well-described.

Trerotola

The Arrow-Trerotola Percutaneous Thrombolytic Device (PTD) (Teleflex Inc.) is a rotating basket used to perform mechanical thrombolysis via clot

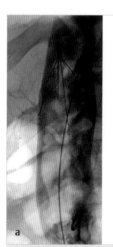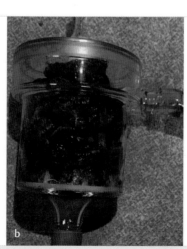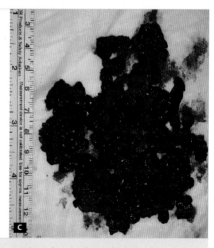

Fig. 7.4 **(a)** Inferior vena cavagram showing large volume, acute-appearing thrombus bridging the indwelling suprarenal inferior vena cava (ICV) filter. **(b)** Fresh thrombus removed within the AngioVac filter. **(c)** Following removal from the filter.

fragmentation. Risks may include device fragmentation, device tip fracture, or separation from the device.[43] The use of the Arrow-Trerotola PTD in the IVC and right atrium have not been well explored in literature.

AngioVac

AngioVac system (Angiodynamics Inc.) is indicated for bulk removal of fresh soft thrombus from vasculature. The 22-Fr AngioVac drainage cannula is passed into the vascular system through a 26-Fr access sheath and once delivered to the area in question, the cannula is connected to a filtered extracorporeal flow circuit. The aspirated blood is driven through the circuit via a standard perfusionist centrifugal pump, filtered of thrombus, and then returned to the vascular system through a 16- to 20-Fr return cannula placed via a separate access site. The process is essentially one of suction thrombectomy but unlike standard guiding catheter suction thrombectomy, the AngioVac does not have the disadvantage of phlebotomy of the patient, since the aspirated blood is returned to the vascular system.

The large diameter of the cannula of the device presents obvious access site issues, but allows for the ready extraction of larger caliber, and even chronic organized thrombotic material. This device can also be applied to both caval and atrial thrombus and should be considered when thrombolysis is contraindicated and/or thrombectomy of the IVC is unsuccessful using smaller caliber devices or in patients with a massive caval clot burden.

AngioJet

The AngioJet system performs thrombectomy via the introduction of a pressurized saline jet stream through the directional orifice in the catheter distal tip, creating an area of localized low pressure via the Venturi effect which draws the thrombus into the adjacent catheter aspiration lumen. The thrombus becomes entrapped and macerated in a process known as rheolysis, with the injected saline and clot particles aspirated into the exhaust lumen of the catheter and out of the body for disposal. This system can also be used as a thrombolytic delivery system, and when activated in the "powerpulse" mode will inject lytic into the thrombus surrounding the catheter tip. The major advantage of the AngioJet rheolytic system is its ability to reduce dose and duration of thrombolytic therapy as a portion of the thrombus removal can be performed mechanically, potentially without lytic infusion.[44] AngioJet has also been successfully used when thrombolytic therapy is absolutely contraindicated, as well as to lyse extensive IVC clots and occluded IVCFs.[45] The newer AngioJet Zelante catheter has been particularly designed for DVT therapy and is especially effective in treating large-diameter veins such as IVC, with its larger directional 8-Fr catheter. However, AngioJet has been linked to some procedure-related complications and deaths have been reported using this device in central venous and PE interventions, thus prompting FDA to issue a black-box warning on the device for use in these areas. This is related to rheolysis-induced hemolysis with subsequent local hyperkalemia and adenosine release which, when it occurs in proximity to cardiac rhythm generators, can lead to significant bradyarrhythmias, ranging from mild bradycardia to asystole. Hemoglobinuria and renal insufficiency are also reported following AngioJet use.[45] A separate observational study revealed that AngioJet is an independent risk factor for acute kidney injury through hemolysis.[46]

Of course, additional thrombectomy devices, which are both purpose-built (Penumbra and others) and off the shelf (directional guiding catheter for suction thrombectomy), exist and are effective to a greater or lesser degree in clot extraction, but an exhaustive discussion of thrombectomy devices is beyond the scope of this chapter.

It is important to note that stand-alone PMT may have limited efficacy and does not consistently remove sufficient thrombus volumes to be clinically significant. It is therefore recommended to combine the CDT and PMT technologies as a "pharmacomechanical" therapy, especially for wall-adherent and large-volume clot burdens often seen in caval thrombosis to achieve optimal clinical success. One study showed that when compared to CDT, pharmacomechanical thrombectomy showed decreased overall interventional treatment time, improved patient outcomes, and reduced hospital costs and intensive care unit (ICU) time.[47,48] Despite the current lack of data, the use of adjunctive mechanical modalities for treating IVC thrombosis in the United States has increased from 16% of treatments in 2005 to 35% in 2011, likely due to increasing recognition of the morbidity associated with IVC thrombosis and the limited effectiveness of traditional anticoagulation.[1]

PTA/Stent (Balloon Expandable/Self-Expanding), Stent Grafts

Despite successful thrombolysis and/or thrombectomy residual caval narrowing may persist. This can be related to either chronic wall adherent thrombus or clot removal-related unmasking of an underlying stenotic lesion. In these instances, adjunctive caval angioplasty and/or stent placement is often needed to reestablish an adequate caval lumen with quality antegrade flow. Percutaneous balloon angioplasty (PTA) can readily compress residual thrombus against the vessel wall during balloon inflation and expand the caval flow channel. There may also be some element of clot maceration with associated surface area increase and subsequent autogenous lysis. Similarly, PTA can expand an underlying stenosing lesion, whether it be malignant or otherwise. Unfortunately, angioplasty often results in only transient caval lumen gain with subsequent elastic recoil. For this reason, angioplasty is often used in combination with stent placement. Additionally, this allows for trapping of thrombotic material between the stent and IVC wall, as well as prevention of elastic recoil.

Not all stents are equal in this regard with various stent constructions simultaneously offering both advantages and disadvantages. The large diameter of the IVC presents the primary challenge when stent placement is considered. Nitinol self-expanding stents offer the benefit of conformability, making them ideal for a kissing configuration extending from the iliac veins into the IVC to treat iliocaval confluence lesions. However, the modest maximal diameter makes this stent type incompatible with single-channel IVC stenting. That said, it is possible to extend the kissing stent configuration cranially from the iliac venous confluence into the IVC for a double barrel lumen when such stents are desired for caval treatment (▶ Fig. 7.5). The interstices of nitinol stents tend to be moderate in size and will trap nonacute thrombus readily, but acute clot will often squeeze through the interstices into the stent lumen in large amounts. Newer, nitinol stents such as Venovo (Bard Peripheral Vascular, Tempe, Arizona) and Vici (Boston Scientific, Marlborough, Massachusetts) offer potential options for large vessel venous stenting; however, their long-term efficacy in comparison to older stents is not yet known. Conversely, Wallstents® (Boston Scientific) are available in large diameters that are suitable for single-channel IVC reconstruction and the woven stent nature results in

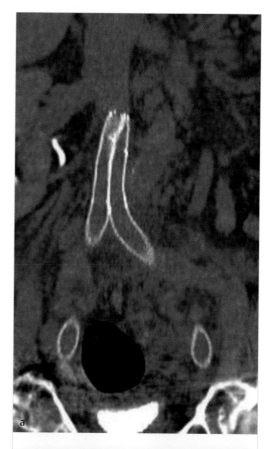

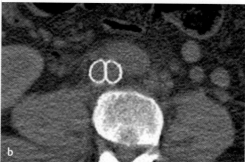

Fig. 7.5 (a) Coronal and (b) axial computed tomography (CT) images of iliocaval nitinol stents extending into the inferior vena cava (IVC) in a double barrel or "kissing" configuration.

small interstices, which readily trap thrombus, even of the acute variety. That said, Wallstents® pose a few challenges including the propensity for these stents to migrate post deployment due to normal IVC motion-induced stent reconfiguration, which over time can result in a "watermelon seeding" effect. This is related to the woven stent design wherein mechanical force applied to one portion of the stent can result in distortion of the stent throughout the device length. This is especially true in the setting of a firm underlying lesion such as a malignant caval stricture. Alternatively, Cook-Z® (Cook Medical, Bloomington, Indiana) stents, designed for endobronchial use, can be deployed in an off-label manner in the IVC. They offer several advantages including large stent size range allowing for single-channel configuration reconstruction, substantial radial force, and wide interstices, which make renal and other vein traversal inconsequential (▶ Fig. 7.6). That said, these same wide interstices make Cook-Z® stents a poor choice for thrombus displacement, acute or chronic. Lastly, balloon expandable stents allow for the greatest lesion

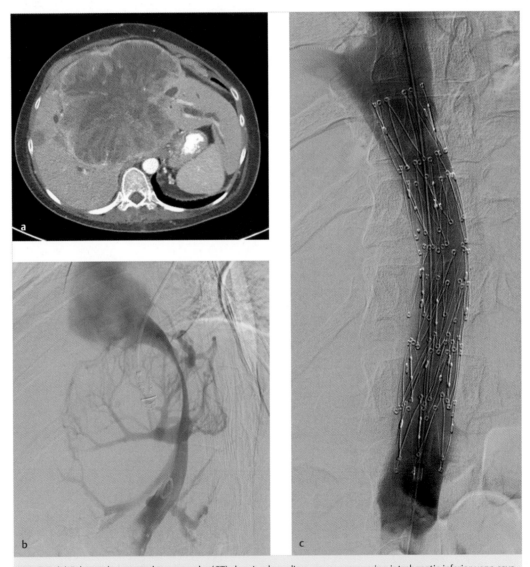

Fig. 7.6 **(a)** Enhanced computed tomography (CT) showing large liver mass compressing intrahepatic inferior vena cava (IVC). **(b)** inferior vena cavagram (IVCgram) showing caval compression and substantial intrahepatic veno-veno collateral flow. **(c)** IVCgram with restored caval patency following overlapping Cook Z stent placement.

expansion capability as well as single-channel reconstruction configuration, but sizing is critical and challenging when using these devices as stent undersizing can lead to subsequent migration (▶ Fig. 7.7). Additionally, care should be taken when using these devices in the setting of IVC thrombus, as lysis of clot trapped between the stent and caval wall following stent placement can result in poor apposition of the stent to the IVC wall with subsequent embolization.

Although specific stent choice may vary between patients for the reasons discussed above, stent placement in general is an effective complement to

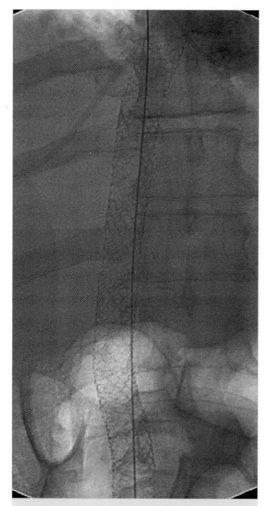

Fig. 7.7 Intraprocedural image with multiple balloon expandable stents bridging the entire suprarenal inferior vena cava (IVC).

thrombolysis, thrombectomy, and angioplasty, as such placement often results in a smooth flow channel with improved caval flow with diminished rates of IVC re-thrombosis,[49] especially in the setting of chronic IVC occlusion.

Further, most IVC thrombotic episodes are identified late in the thrombosis course resulting in a combination of acute soft thrombus and chronic fibrotic thrombus at presentation. In most cases, the acute thrombus component will readily lyse with standard pharmacologic and mechanical techniques. The chronic thrombotic component, however, is less amenable to either thrombolysis or thrombectomy therapy[1] making stent placement a common occurrence in caval therapy.

Finally, stent-grafts have been widely used in situations that require additional reinforcement and rupture containment with some consideration for their use in preventing recurrent stenosis. Such devices have been successfully used in the venous system to treat dialysis access venous outflow lesions, as well as in the setting of traumatic IVC and other large vein injuries. However, stent graft efficacy in treating IVC thrombosis has not been validated and should therefore be reserved for select cases. Piffaretti et al have noted that IVC endovascular aneurysm repair (EVAR) is associated with risks of progressive IVC narrowing, re-thrombosis, and pulmonary embolization.[50] The potential risks of using stent-grafts to treat IVC thrombosis are primarily related to challenges with graft sizing and the likelihood for graft thrombosis.

7.5.2 Chronic IVC Thrombosis

Wire/Catheter

Although the abovementioned reconstructive techniques are usually quite successful in restoring caval patency and relieving associated symptoms, traversal of the occluded IVC segment is often the most challenging part of the procedure. Certainly, if guidewire traversal is unsuccessful then a technical failure occurs. Although crossing fresh caval thrombus is generally quite simple, the presence of an underlying stenotic lesion can make the traversal substantially more challenging as the stenosing lesion may be obscured by the superimposed fresh clot. In these instances, clot lysis or thrombectomy prior to lesion traversal is preferred as the lesion can then be clearly visualized, mapped, and crossed in a more typical manner (▶ Fig. 7.8). That said, the presence of an underlying lesion is often not known until after the

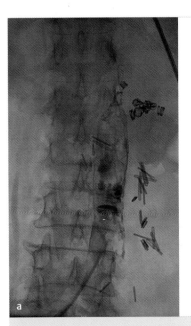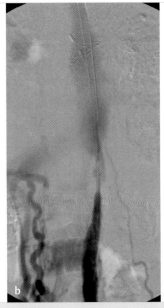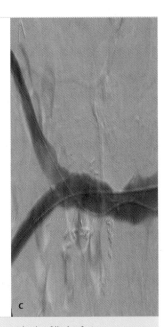

Fig. 7.8 (a) Inferior vena cavagram (IVCgram) prior to thrombolysis/thrombectomy with clot-filled inferior vena cava (IVC) and no obvious focal lesion. **(b)** Repeat IVCgram following clot removal reveals a focal underlying high-grade stenosis. **(c)** Caval patency following angioplasty and kissing stent placement.

caval thrombus has been removed. This scenario is quite different than that encountered in traversal of chronic clot, which in most cases is substantially more challenging than traversal of acute clot. Additionally, in the setting of longstanding caval thrombosis, some degree of venous sclerosis with secondary IVC narrowing can occur that at times can progress to complete caval obliteration. In this instance, extensive collaterals are usually present, and their opacification can obscure any small residual IVC channel making targeting of the true lumen even more challenging. Historically, chronic IVC occlusions of this type were managed only surgically, with poor long-term results[51] and little role for endovascular management. However, the advent of the enhanced guidewires, catheters, crossing systems, and specialized devices has reduced the proportion of untraversable, chronic, total IVC occlusions substantially.

When planning a caval occlusion procedure, the first important step is the selection of proper access site(s). In the setting of fresh thrombus, a single access site is usually adequate for procedure performance. The access is ideally chosen to allow for antegrade, rather than retrograde, traversal of the IVC. Such traversal is in the direction of normal blood flow, allowing for better contrast opacification via catheter/sheath injection, as opposed to the retrograde traversal and subsequent retrograde contrast injection. Additionally, an antegrade access allows the operator to assess caval inflow, since it is an important element in determining treatment durability. Depending on inflow vessel patency, femoral, popliteal, or tibial vein access can be used. Given the relatively larger IVC lumen size and the associated larger treatment device caliber, the largest inflow vessel that can be accessed should be chosen, with preference for access vessel patency. This principle is somewhat expanded when dealing with chronic thrombus, as multiple access sites are often needed in these cases. Specifically, plan should be made to allow for placement of a targeting device, such as a loop snare, at the cephalad end of the chronic occlusion length to optimize likelihood of successful reentry into the true lumen.

Once the access site has been selected, the access sheath must be chosen. Although the targeting sheath size merely needs to be large enough to accommodate the targeting device utilized, selection of the crossing sheath is far more nuanced. One needs to consider not only sheath diameter, but also length, stiffness, directionality, and compatibility with potential devices to be used and coaxial systems deployed. Sheath length should be chosen to allow for the sheath tip to reach central to the caudal end of the occlusion. This allows for sheath stiffening of the crossing system and advancement of the sheath into the caudal end of the occlusion for increased stability and diminished likelihood of crossing device buckling in the patent venous segment below the occlusion during advancement. Along with length, sheath stiffness is also an important consideration. A stiffer sheath will allow for more stability during device advancement, but sheath stiffness can also have a negative attribute. An extremely stiff sheath can make the crossing system too rigid, not allowing to flex, thus increasing the likelihood of IVC wall penetration and extraluminal passage. Further, such a sheath can inadvertently force the crossing system to approach the IVC occlusion at an inopportune angle, rather than directly in line with the caval wall. To this end, sheath directionality can be a valuable attribute in occlusion traversal. A curved or angled sheath tip can allow for manipulation of the occlusion approach angle and subsequent improved linearity and column strength of the crossing system. Finally, pre-procedure planning and subsequent sheath selection should account for appropriate entry sheath diameter so that it would fit all potential devices to be used. Specifically, when consideration is given to potential coaxial, triaxial, or multiaxial system use with multiple sheaths or guiding catheters placed, the compatibility of these devices with one another and with the initial access sheath should be considered.

Following sheath selection and attainment of planned accesses, choosing the guidewire and catheter for lesion crossing is of paramount importance. The important characteristics for consideration in guidewire selection include tip load, tip and shaft stiffness, flexibility, shape manipulation ability, shaping memory, and steerability.[52] There are two broad types of guidewires available, hydrophilic and nonhydrophilic. Hydrophilic guidewires provide good maneuverability and lubricity and can be advanced with minimal resistance, even through thrombus, and may be steered easily despite access vessel angulation.[52] This characteristic makes hydrophilic wires the device of choice for caval occlusion traversal. However, their gliding capability increases the possibility of intramural or transmural passage and care should be taken to ensure the advancing wire is moving along the expected path of the IVC lumen.

Similar to the variability seen with guidewires, the associated catheters also have specific characteristics that affect performance. As a rule, catheter selection considerations are comparable to those used in sheath selection. The most frequently considered of these include catheter taper, directionality, stiffness, and hydrophilia. Catheter taper is an especially important consideration in the setting of chronic caval occlusion as a nontapered catheter may not track over the crossing guidewire following successful traversal. Recanalization is generally approached by gradually stiffening the system through use of different guidewire, catheter, guiding catheter, and guiding sheath combinations to allow for progressively greater force delivery at the wire tip. However, it has been shown that the tactile feel of the guidewire decreases as stiffness of the tip increases.[53]

Special Devices

Advanced Crossing Techniques— Guidewire Back End and Needles

In the rare instance where a progressively stiffened multiaxial system will not allow for caval occlusion traversal, consideration can be given to the use of advanced crossing techniques including guidewire back end, sheathed needle passage, and radiofrequency (RF) energy assisted wire traversal. The least penetrating of these techniques is to use the back end of a guidewire, usually hydrophilic, either in a straight or clamp modified directional form, through the preexisting multiaxial system. This technique is meant to create a new passage within the occlusion through which the front end of the guidewire is subsequently manipulated rather than advancing the guidewire back end through the entire occlusion length.

The next most penetrating technique involves the use of a styletted needle with a modified (bent) tip for steerability. This needle, which must be long enough to traverse the entire lesion length, is advanced through the vascular system to the lesion with fluoroscopic guidance along the entire path and through a protective sheath, preferably wire-supported, to decrease the likelihood of needle penetration through the sheath wall. Once appropriately positioned at the lesion location, the needle is then advanced through the occlusion length and engaged by the targeting device. The stylet is removed, and the guidewire is passed through the needle, engaging the targeting device.

Alternatively, a sheathed or catheter associated needle can be used in a similar manner.

RF Wire

Finally, the RF energy guidewire offers the greatest degree of penetrating ability. This device uses a length-calibrated, directional wire connected to an RF generator to deliver RF energy to the wire tip which in turn vaporizes a channel through the occlusions. The energized wire will pass readily through any noncalcified soft tissue, so extraordinary care must be taken during use. Passage into adjacent critical structures, such as bowel, pancreas, and aorta, is a very realistic outcome, if accurate targeting is not performed. Caution aside, the RF wire allows for successful occlusion traversal when all other techniques have failed. It has been shown that RF wire is an efficient procedure in treating symptomatic, chronic central vein occlusions when conventional endovascular techniques have failed.[54] Given the increased risks associated with the advanced occlusion transversal techniques, they should be reserved for patients with substantial occlusion-related symptoms in whom the risk/benefit ratio for the procedure is deemed appropriate.

Occlusion Traversal Navigation Devices

In addition to targeting described above, additional traversal navigation specificity can be obtained using intraprocedural intravascular ultrasound (IVUS) and cone-beam CT. Targeting is often performed to ensure accurate positioning of catheters, wires, and other treatment modalities. A target, such as a loop snare, is placed into the desired venous location and is used as physical target to aim traversal devices and thereby facilitate occlusion traversal.

IVUS can provide useful complementary information about traversal device location within the lumen, relative to the occlusion. IVUS allows for unaffected viewing angle, thereby providing a clearer and more accurate diagnostic picture. That said, in the venous system, IVUS is more often used in aiding stent placement accuracy, vessel sizing, and determining adequacy of lumen gain after treatment rather than in primary lesion traversal.

Conversely, cone-beam CT is extraordinarily valuable in guiding traversal, as it allows for device location in three dimensions, compared to two-dimensional X-ray. Additionally, cone-beam CT is helpful in imaging of traversal device position relative to that of critical adjacent structures and can be undertaken repeatedly during device advancement allowing for more accurate localization and safety.

7.5.3 Right Atrial Interventions

In situ or embolized RA thrombi are considered to be of considerable risk given the possibility of progressive enlargement and/or embolization to the pulmonary vasculature. Hence, current management strategy for RA thrombus remains an area of uncertainty.

Catheter-Directed Thrombolysis (CDT)

Similar to IVC thrombus, dissolution of RA clot with catheter-directed thrombolytic infusion can be successful when the thrombus is acute in nature, but much less so in the setting of chronic thrombotic material. During lytic therapy, there is a substantial risk of clot fragmentation and pulmonary embolization. Thus, atrial thrombolytic therapy should be used with caution.[55]

It is important to understand there are no current guidelines that address CDT as an option for RA thrombosis. However, the authors believe CDT is a valuable option for treating patients with this challenging diagnosis.

When associated with intracardiac devices, atrial thrombus carries an especially high risk for fragmentation and embolization during device extraction.[57] In this setting, a course of thrombolysis prior to implanted device extraction may reduce the potential embolized clot burden. However, unlike free-floating right heart thrombi which most frequently arise from the lower extremity veins and may be either acute or chronic in nature, device-associated thrombi are more often chronic and therefore less apt to respond to lysis.[55] In a case described by Gawaz et al,[56] as well as others, a successful thrombolytic therapy with standard transvenous lead extraction can be used to reduce the thrombus burden in order to avoid massive PE.[56]

Thrombectomy
Suction Thrombectomy

In the setting of unsuccessful lysis, or of thrombolytic contraindication, or as an augment to lysis, atrial thrombectomy can be undertaken. A variety of thrombectomy techniques are available, each of which offers advantages and disadvantage in this setting, primarily related to the large size of the atrium and to the delicate nature of the chamber and constituents. The options for atrial thrombectomy can include both suction and mechanical devices. Suction thrombectomy can be performed in a variety of different ways using a range of devices.

Guiding Catheter

At the simplest level, wide-orifice directional guiding catheters can be used as a crude means for atrial suction thrombectomy. The guiding catheter tip is advanced near the clot, most likely under direct TEE guidance, the guidewire removed, and negative pressure applied by suctioning through a large syringe at the guiding catheter hub resulting in aspiration of contents adjacent to the catheter tip into the catheter. In cases where the clot is trapped in the catheter orifice by the suction, but cannot be aspirated through the entire catheter lumen, the catheter can be withdrawn while maintaining negative pressure with continued syringe aspiration thereby drawing the thrombus out from the atrium. Similar challenges may be noted as the guiding catheter is drawn into the associated vascular sheath if the sheath diameter is not adequate to accept the clot. When successful, this leads to immediate thrombus load reduction in the RA. The advantages of this technique are ease of use and employment of widely available, inexpensive equipment.

Penumbra Aspiration System

A specialized guiding catheter thrombectomy system, the Penumbra aspiration system has been used effectively for suction thrombectomy, in which emboli and thrombi are removed from vessels through continuous negative suction, while allowing for rapid restoration of blood flow. The Penumbra guiding catheters are specifically designed for clot extraction with wide lumen and ready trackability. Additionally, the system employs a continuous negative suction generated by a specialized vacuum generator, theoretically creating a more effective and more consistent suctioning force. Although useful for clot extraction in peripheral vasculature as well as intracranially, in the authors' experience, this system has limited large vessel utility due to the substantial blood loss that occurs during negative pressure suction in large caliber vascular structures, such as the atria.

AngioJet Rheolytic Thrombectomy

As previously discussed, the AngioJet rheolytic thrombectomy has been linked to some procedure-related complications and deaths have been reported using this device in PE interventions prompting FDA to issue a black-box warning on the device for use in such a central location. Due to safety concerns, the AngioJet device should not be used to treat RA thrombus as substantial bradyarrhythmia and possibly asystole are likely outcomes.

AngioVac System

Of considerable interest is the AngioVac system which is indicated for bulk removal of fresh soft thrombus from vasculature. As discussed earlier, AngioVac does not have the disadvantage of phlebotomy of the patient, as the aspirated blood is returned to the vascular system. One single-center study showed successful partial or complete clot abatement in seven consecutive patients presenting with large central thrombi, including in the right atrium, using the AngioVac device.[58] A separate study demonstrated effective complete en bloc AngioVac removal of an RA thrombus.[59] A retrospective analysis of AngioVac thrombectomy found that procedural success was achieved in 4/6 (67%) RA masses/thrombi.[60] The large diameter of the device cannula presents obvious access site hemostasis issues, but it allows for the ready extraction of larger caliber, chronic, organized thrombotic material. In the authors' opinion, the AngioVac system is the preferred thrombectomy device for atrial clot extraction.

Mechanical Thrombectomy

Rotational devices, such as the Cleaner or the Trerotola system, offer a theoretical benefit of clot fragmentation and subsequent improved extraction ability, but this must be balanced against dangers of thrombus fragment distal PE and concern for valve or chordae entanglement. Serious consideration should be given prior to their use in the atrium given the potential for serious adverse events.

7.6 Conclusion

IVC thrombosis and RA thrombosis are both less prevalent, high morbidity and mortality subsets of

DVT. Due to the variability in presentation of both RA and IVC thromboses, the exact annual prevalence of these diseases remains elusive.

Diagnosis of both IVC and RA thromboses can be challenging at times due to the nonspecific presentations. In patients with leg DVT in whom there are additional signs or symptoms suggestive of possible iliocaval thrombosis, a contrast-enhanced CT should be performed. In case of RA thrombosis, atrial filling defects are on occasion identified; however, these findings are typically indistinct secondary to cardiac motion, despite utilization of cardiac gating technique. Such findings should be followed up by more detailed imaging via TEE.

Once diagnosis is made, immediate clinical treatment is warranted to avoid acute and chronic complications. The limited effectiveness of anticoagulation alone, and the decreased precision and complications associated with systemic thrombolysis therapy, has led to development of numerous targeted endovascular therapies. CDT is a modality of choice for dissolving an acute clot and may be used in combination with other thrombolytic methods. Due to the risk of hemorrhagic complications during CDT, PMT devices have emerged as an advantageous option for the treatment of acute DVT.

Although the above-mentioned techniques are usually successful in restoring caval patency and relieving associated symptoms in acute thrombosis, traversal of the chronically occluded IVC segment is often more challenging and requires use of advanced crossing techniques and devices. Due to the absence of published trials and societal guidelines, a careful selection of the targeted technique is essential for successful endovascular management of IVC and RA thromboses.

References

[1] Alkhouli M, Morad M, Narins CR, Raza F, Bashir R. Inferior vena cava thrombosis. JACC Cardiovasc Interv. 2016; 9(7): 629–643

[2] Agnelli G, Verso M, Ageno W, et al. MASTER investigators. The MASTER registry on venous thromboembolism: description of the study cohort. Thromb Res. 2008; 121(5):605–610

[3] McAree BJ, O'Donnell ME, Fitzmaurice GJ, Reid JA, Spence RA, Lee B. Inferior vena cava thrombosis: a review of current practice. Vasc Med. 2013; 18(1):32–43

[4] Kahn SR. The post-thrombotic syndrome: the forgotten morbidity of deep venous thrombosis. J Thromb Thrombolysis. 2006; 21(1):41–48

[5] Martin MJ, Blair KS, Curry TK, Singh N. Vena cava filters: current concepts and controversies for the surgeon. Curr Probl Surg. 2010; 47(7):524–618

[6] Milovanovic L, Kennedy SA, Midia M. Procedural and indwelling complications with inferior vena cava filters: frequency, etiology, and management. Semin Intervent Radiol. 2015; 32 (1):34–41

[7] Casazza F, Bongarzoni A, Centonze F, Morpurgo M. Prevalence and prognostic significance of right-sided cardiac mobile thrombi in acute massive pulmonary embolism. Am J Cardiol. 1997; 79(10):1433–1435

[8] Goldhaber SZ, Visani L, De Rosa M. Acute pulmonary embolism: clinical outcomes in the International Cooperative Pulmonary Embolism Registry (ICOPER). Lancet. 1999; 353 (9162):1386–1389

[9] Gilon D, Schechter D, Rein AJ, et al. Right atrial thrombi are related to indwelling central venous catheter position: insights into time course and possible mechanism of formation. Am Heart J. 1998; 135(3):457–462

[10] Sitwala PS, Ladia VM, Brahmbhatt PB, Jain V, Bajaj K. Inferior vena cava anomaly: a risk for deep vein thrombosis. N Am J Med Sci. 2014; 6(11):601–603

[11] Chuang VP, Mena CE, Hoskins PA. Congenital anomalies of the inferior vena cava. Review of embryogenesis and presentation of a simplified classification. Br J Radiol. 1974; 47 (556):206–213

[12] Chee YL, Culligan DJ, Watson HG. Inferior vena cava malformation as a risk factor for deep venous thrombosis in the young. Br J Haematol. 2001; 114(4):878–880

[13] Felner JM, Churchwell AL, Murphy DA. Right atrial thromboemboli: clinical, echocardiographic and pathophysiologic manifestations. J Am Coll Cardiol. 1984; 4(5):1041–1051

[14] Dahlbäck B. Advances in understanding pathogenic mechanisms of thrombophilic disorders. Blood. 2008; 112(1):19–27

[15] De Stefano V, Martinelli I, Mannucci PM, et al. The risk of recurrent deep venous thrombosis among heterozygous carriers of both factor V Leiden and the G20210A prothrombin mutation. N Engl J Med. 1999; 341(11):801–806

[16] Poort SR, Rosendaal FR, Reitsma PH, Bertina RM. A common genetic variation in the 3′-untranslated region of the prothrombin gene is associated with elevated plasma prothrombin levels and an increase in venous thrombosis. Blood. 1996; 88(10): 3698–3703

[17] Miletich J, Sherman L, Broze G, Jr. Absence of thrombosis in subjects with heterozygous protein C deficiency. N Engl J Med. 1987; 317(16):991–996

[18] Lentz SR. Mechanisms of homocysteine-induced atherothrombosis. J Thromb Haemost. 2005; 3(8):1646–1654

[19] Lovecchio F. Heparin-induced thrombocytopenia. Clin Toxicol (Phila). 2014; 52(6):579–583

[20] Forauer AR, Theoharis C. Histologic changes in the human vein wall adjacent to indwelling central venous catheters. J Vasc Interv Radiol. 2003; 14(9 Pt 1):1163–1168

[21] Verso M, Agnelli G. Venous thromboembolism associated with long-term use of central venous catheters in cancer patients. J Clin Oncol. 2003; 21(19):3665–3675

[22] Prandoni P, Polistena P, Bernardi E, et al. Upper-extremity deep vein thrombosis. Risk factors, diagnosis, and complications. Arch Intern Med. 1997; 157(1):57–62

[23] Fallouh N, McGuirk HM, Flanders SA, Chopra V. Peripherally inserted central catheter-associated deep vein thrombosis: a narrative review. Am J Med. 2015; 128(7):722–738

[24] Molvar C. Inferior vena cava filtration in the management of venous thromboembolism: filtering the data. Semin Intervent Radiol. 2012; 29(3):204–217

[25] Carrier M, Lazo-Langner A, Shivakumar S, et al. SOME Investigators. Screening for occult cancer in unprovoked venous thromboembolism. N Engl J Med. 2015; 373(8):697–704

[26] Deso SE, Idakoji IA, Kuo WT. Evidence-based evaluation of inferior vena cava filter complications based on filter type. Semin Intervent Radiol. 2016; 33(2):93–100

[27] Corriere MA, Sauve KJ, Ayerdi J, et al. Vena cava filters and inferior vena cava thrombosis. J Vasc Surg. 2007; 45(4):789–794

[28] Vongpatanasin W, Hillis LD, Lange RA. Prosthetic heart valves. N Engl J Med. 1996; 335(6):407–416

[29] Habib G, Hoen B, Tornos P, et al. ESC Committee for Practice Guidelines, Endorsed by the European Society of Clinical Microbiology and Infectious Diseases (ESCMID) and the International Society of Chemotherapy (ISC) for Infection and Cancer. Guidelines on the prevention, diagnosis, and treatment of infective endocarditis (new version 2009): the Task Force on the Prevention, Diagnosis, and Treatment of Infective Endocarditis of the European Society of Cardiology (ESC). Eur Heart J. 2009; 30(19):2369–2413

[30] Kandpal H, Sharma R, Gamangatti S, Srivastava DN, Vashisht S. Imaging the inferior vena cava: a road less traveled. Radiographics. 2008; 28(3):669–689

[31] Pillari G, Kumari S, Phillips G, Cruz V, Pochaczevsky R, Marc J. Computed tomography in ileofemoral venous thrombosis: extension to inferior vena cava defined with foot vein infusion. J Comput Assist Tomogr. 1981; 5(3):375–377

[32] Thompson CA, Skelton TN. Thromboembolism in the right side of the heart. South Med J. 1999; 92(8):826–830

[33] Chapoutot L, Nazeyrollas P, Metz D, et al. Floating right heart thrombi and pulmonary embolism: diagnosis, outcome and therapeutic management. Cardiology. 1996; 87(2):169–174

[34] Kearon C, Akl EA, Ornelas J, et al. Antithrombotic therapy for VTE disease: CHEST guideline and expert panel report. Chest. 2016; 149(2):315–352

[35] Uchino K, Hernandez AV. Dabigatran association with higher risk of acute coronary events: meta-analysis of noninferiority randomized controlled trials. Arch Intern Med. 2012; 172(5):397–402

[36] Wang X, Chen Z, Cai Q. Catheter-directed thrombolysis for double inferior vena cava with deep venous thrombosis: a case report and literature review. Phlebology. 2014; 29(7):480–483

[37] Khan JU, Takemoto CM, Casella JF, Streiff MB, Nwankwo IJ, Kim HS. Catheter-directed thrombolysis of inferior vena cava thrombosis in a 13-day-old neonate and review of literature. Cardiovasc Intervent Radiol. 2008; 31 Suppl 2:S153–S160

[38] Bookstein JJ, Bookstein FL. Pulse-spray thrombolysis with reteplase: optimization and comparison with tPA in a rabbit model. J Vasc Interv Radiol. 2001; 12(11):1319–1324

[39] Razavi MK, Wong H, Kee ST, Sze DY, Semba CP, Dake MD. Initial clinical results of tenecteplase (TNK) in catheter-directed thrombolytic therapy. J Endovasc Ther. 2002; 9(5):593–598

[40] Yuksel A, Tuydes O. Midterm outcomes of pharmacomechanical thrombectomy in the treatment of lower extremity deep vein thrombosis with a rotational thrombectomy device. Vasc Endovasc Surg. 2017; 51(5):301–306

[41] Calik ES, Dag O, Kaygin MA, Onk OA, Erkut B. Pharmacomechanical thrombectomy for acute symptomatic lower extremity deep venous thrombosis. Heart Surg Forum. 2015; 18(4):E178–E183

[42] Köksoy C, Yilmaz MF, Başbuğ HS, et al. Pharmacomechanical thrombolysis of symptomatic acute and subacute deep vein thrombosis with a rotational thrombectomy device. J Vasc Interv Radiol. 2014; 25(12):1895–1900

[43] Dupaix R, Mohan PP. Trerotola device fragmentation. Cardiovasc Intervent Radiol. 2017; 40(4):636–638

[44] Kuo WT, Gould MK, Louie JD, Rosenberg JK, Sze DY, Hofmann LV. Catheter-directed therapy for the treatment of massive pulmonary embolism: systematic review and meta-analysis of modern techniques. J Vasc Interv Radiol. 2009; 20(11):1431–1440

[45] Dwarka D, Schwartz SA, Smyth SH, O'Brien MJ. Bradyarrhythmias during use of the AngioJet system. J Vasc Interv Radiol. 2006; 17(10):1693–1695

[46] Escobar GA, Burks D, Abate MR, et al. Risk of acute kidney injury after percutaneous pharmacomechanical thrombectomy using AngioJet in venous and arterial thrombosis. Ann Vasc Surg. 2017; 42:238–245

[47] Bush RL, Lin PH, Bates JT, Mureebe L, Zhou W, Lumsden AB. Pharmacomechanical thrombectomy for treatment of symptomatic lower extremity deep venous thrombosis: safety and feasibility study. J Vasc Surg. 2004; 40(5):965–970

[48] Lin PH, Zhou W, Dardik A, et al. Catheter-direct thrombolysis versus pharmacomechanical thrombectomy for treatment of symptomatic lower extremity deep venous thrombosis. Am J Surg. 2006; 192(6):782–788

[49] Chick JFB, Jo A, Meadows JM, et al. Endovascular iliocaval stent reconstruction for inferior vena cava filter-associated iliocaval thrombosis: approach, technical success, safety, and two-year outcomes in 120 patients. J Vasc Interv Radiol. 2017; 28(7):933–939

[50] Piffaretti G, Carrafiello G, Piacentino F, Castelli P. Traumatic IVC injury and repair: the endovascular alternative. Endovascular Today. 2013(November):39–44

[51] Garg N, Gloviczki P, Karimi KM, et al. Factors affecting outcome of open and hybrid reconstructions for nonmalignant obstruction of iliofemoral veins and inferior vena cava. J Vasc Surg. 2011; 53(2):383–393

[52] Ge JB. Current status of percutaneous coronary intervention of chronic total occlusion. J Zhejiang Univ Sci B. 2012; 13(8):589–602

[53] Dave B. Recanalization of chronic total occlusion lesions: a critical appraisal of current devices and techniques. J Clin Diagn Res. 2016; 10(9):OE01–OE07

[54] Guimaraes M, Schonholz C, Hannegan C, Anderson MB, Shi J, Selby B, Jr. Radiofrequency wire for the recanalization of central vein occlusions that have failed conventional endovascular techniques. J Vasc Interv Radiol. 2012; 23(8):1016–1021

[55] Starkey IR, de Bono DP. Echocardiographic identification of right-sided cardiac intracavitary thromboembolus in massive pulmonary embolism. Circulation. 1982; 66(6):1322–1325

[56] Mueller KA, Mueller II, Weig HJ, Doernberger V, Gawaz M. Thrombolysis is an appropriate treatment in lead-associated infective endocarditis with giant vegetations located on the right atrial lead. BMJ Case Rep. 2012 Jun 14;2012:bcr0920114855. doi: 10.1136/bcr.09.2011.4855. PMID: 22707697; PMCID: PMC3387473.

[57] Rose PS, Punjabi NM, Pearse DB. Treatment of right heart thromboemboli. Chest. 2002; 121(3):806–814

[58] Resnick SA, O'Brien D, Strain D, et al. Single-center experience using AngioVac with extracorporeal bypass for mechanical thrombectomy of atrial and central vein thrombi. J Vasc Interv Radiol. 2016; 27(5):723–729.e1

[59] Dudiy Y, Kronzon I, Cohen HA, Ruiz CE. Vacuum thrombectomy of large right atrial thrombus. Catheter Cardiovasc Interv. 2012; 79(2):344–347

[60] Moriarty JM, Al-Hakim R, Bansal A, Park JK. Removal of caval and right atrial thrombi and masses using the AngioVac device: initial operative experience. J Vasc Interv Radiol. 2016; 27(10):1584–1591

Chapter 8

Interventional Approaches to Recanalization of Chronic Central Venous Occlusions

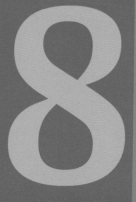

8 Interventional Approaches to Recanalization of Chronic Central Venous Occlusions

Shaun W. McLaughlin, Loren Mead, and Deepak Sudheendra

Keywords: recanalization, central venous occlusion

8.1 Introduction

Thromboembolic venous disease affects nearly a million people per year in the United States in the form of deep vein thrombosis (DVT) or pulmonary embolism (PE), and is estimated to be a leading cause of death.[1] DVT comprises the majority of venous thromboembolic events and management is clear in the acute setting where widely accepted guidelines advise a course of anticoagulation (AC) therapy, or placement of an inferior vena cava (IVC) filter in those not suitable for AC. However, the incidence of recurrence is estimated to be nearly 30% after a prior proximal DVT.[2] Those with multiple risk factors, such as obesity, recent hospitalization, and venous insufficiency, are susceptible to more complex disease presentation where chronic total occlusion (CTO) of the central venous system can occur and the optimal management strategy is less clear.[3,4]

In patients with recurrent, multisegmental thrombosis, particularly those with iliofemoral and iliocaval involvement, interventional therapies such as catheter-directed thrombolysis (CDT) and pharmacomechanical thrombectomy, combined with venoplasty and stenting of underlying stenoses, has become the standard of care where systemic AC alone has failed.[5] In the case of central CTO, when there is an inability to cross a lesion using conventional techniques, operator experience and resources may be lacking if not properly prepared prior to intervention. Significant endovascular expertise and experience is essential in treating patients with complex severe chronic venous disease and it is our goal here to set the operator up for success when undertaking these often lengthy, but rewarding procedures.

Recanalization of central CTO possesses unique challenges not faced in the acute setting. In the chronic setting, the choice of instruments, interventional approaches, patient preparation, and outcomes differs. The commonly accepted definition of a chronic versus acute thrombosis is whether the clot has been > 28 days.[6] With central CTOs, the majority of patients present > 1 month after the initial event when symptoms of postthrombotic syndrome (PTS) have had time to manifest themselves. For this discussion, central venous occlusions are defined as occlusions that occur within the iliac veins, IVC, subclavian vein, brachiocephalic vein, and superior vena cava (SVC), and will focus mainly on recanalization of the lower venous system. Compared to distal venous occlusions, which are more easily compensated by collateralization to the deep femoral vein and superficial veins, occlusions of the iliac and caval segments have poorer chances of sufficient collateralization and often result in PTS.[7] Endovascular recanalization and stent placement can improve outflow obstruction and has replaced open surgery in the initial treatment of CTOs of the iliac veins and IVC. Procedural success rates in recanalization of a central CTO has ranged from 83 to 95%. However, long-term patency in occlusive lesions remains 10 to 20% less than that for stenotic lesions caused by external compression from tumors or congenital venous abnormalities such as May–Thurner syndrome.[8] These data support the notion that patients with complete thrombotic obstruction of the iliocaval venous segment are a different population than those with stenotic obstructions and should be treated differently.

The development of clot over time in the central venous system leads to increased ambulatory venous pressures in the lower extremities and subsequently significant venous insufficiency and chronic venous disorders. Standardization of the definition of chronic venous disorders was developed in 1994 by an ad hoc committee of the American Venous Forum.[9] Out of this forum came the CEAP (clinical, etiological, anatomy, and pathophysiology) classification, which has become adopted worldwide to facilitate meaningful communication about CVD and serve as a basis for managing patients and tracking clinical outcomes (▶ Table 8.1).

Many authors have accepted the CEAP classification along with the Venous Clinical Severity Score (VCSS) to assess treatment outcomes.[10] The VCSS was instituted in response to the CEAP system not

Table 8.1 The 2020 update to the CEAP (clinical, etiological, anatomy, and pathophysiology) classification

C_5	Healed
C_6	Active venous ulcer
C_{6r}	Recurrent active venous ulcer
Etiologic classification (E)	
E_p	Primary
E_s	Secondary
E_{si}	Secondary—intravenous
E_{se}	Secondary—extravenous
E_c	Congenital
E_n	No cause identified
Anatomic classification (A)	
A_s	Superficial
A_d	Deep
A_p	Perforator
A_n	No venous anatomic location identified
Pathophysiologic classification (P)	
P_r	Reflux
P_o	Obstruction
P_{ro}	Reflux and obstruction
P_n	No pathology identified

Source: *Seminars in Interventional Radiology Vol. 38 No. 2/2021.*

depicting fully the spectrum of the severity of venous disease.[11,12] This scoring system was designed to be responsive to disease progression and changes in the severity over time (▶ Table 8.2). These tools were originally developed for guiding interventions for treating venous insufficiency; however, they have proven to be translatable to treatment of chronic venous occlusions. The clinical course of both entities eventually leads to the same form of disability for the patients involved. These grading systems have become the standard of care when reporting outcomes in treating venous disease, and interventionalists should be familiar with these systems when charting and reporting outcomes.

One of the most significant complications of long-standing CTO of the central venous system is PTS. At least one in every two to three patients with DVT will develop PTS and one-third to one-half of the patients will develop PTS after an acute episode of proximal DVT despite AC.[13] Pain, swelling, stasis pigmentation, and venous ectasia of the leg secondary to venous obstruction and perivenous inflammation are minor signs of early symptomatic PTS. In severe cases of proximal DVT, life-threatening phlegmasia cerulea dolens may result due to ischemia and gangrene of the extremity. With significant clot burden, fatal pulmonary embolus can occur due to clot migrating from the lower extremity to the pulmonary circulation. In time, chronic venous hypertension will result in persistent venous obstruction and damage to the venous valves. Once these changes occur, a cascade of sequelae are likely to develop including chronic edema → fibrin deposition in the interstitial soft tissues → poor oxygen exchange and skin changes → painful inflammation of the lower extremity → therapy resistant ulcers.[14,15] CTOs often also lead to extensive collateral formation to bypass the occluded segments of the iliocaval system and often these collaterals are visible on physical examination (▶ Fig. 8.1). These changes have been correlated to ambulatory venous pressures.[16] Pressures of < 28 mm Hg are normally asymptomatic, but at 36 mm Hg varicosities are visible. Edema and hyperpigmentation occur in the 41 to 47 mm Hg range and ulceration occurs at around 60 mm Hg. Therefore, the greater the ambulatory venous pressure, the worse the symptoms of PTS. Thrombus removal in severe cases is therefore critical and it has been shown that early thrombus removal leads to a lower incidence of symptoms related to PTS.[17,18]

Recently, the Villalta scoring system for PTS, which overcomes some of the limitations associated with VCSS and CEAP classification, has been described.[19] This scoring system was specifically designed for patients with chronic venous occlusive disease in mind, and it encompasses the vast majority of clinical scenarios that are encountered. In 2008, the International Society on Thrombosis and Haemostasis in Vienna recommended that this scoring system be used for the diagnosis and grading of PTS in clinical trials.[20] When combined with a venous-specific quality of life questionnaire, the Villalta score can be considered the "gold standard" for diagnosis, classification, and monitoring interventions for PTS in patients with CTOs.

Table 8.2 Venous clinical severity score, 2010 revision (VCSS-R) worksheet

Attribute	Absent = 0		Mild = 1		Moderate = 2		Severe = 3	
Pain or other discomfort (i.e., aching, heaviness, fatigue, soreness, burning)	None		Occasional, not restricting daily activities		Interferes but does not prevent regular daily activities		Limits most regular daily activities	
	Rt	Lt	Rt	Lt	Rt	Lt	Rt	Lt
Varicose veins ≥3 mm diameter in the standing position	None		Few: (also corona phlebectatica)		Calf *or* thigh		Calf and thigh	
	Rt	Lt	Rt	Lt	Rt	Lt	Rt	Lt
Venous edema	None		Foot and ankle		Above the ankle and below the knee		To the knee and above the knee	
	Rt	Lt	Rt	Lt	Rt	Lt	Rt	Lt
Skin pigmentation	None or focal		Perimalleolar		Lower third of the calf		Above the lower third of the calf	
	Rt	Lt	Rt	Lt	Rt	Lt	Rt	Lt
Inflammation Erythema, cellulitis, venous eczema, and dermatitis	None		Perimalleolar		Lower third of the calf		Above the lower third of the calf	
	Rt	Lt	Rt	Lt	Rt	Lt	Rt	Lt
Induration Chronic edema, atrophie blanche, lipodermatosclerosis	None		Perimalleolar		Lower third of the calf		Above the lower third of the calf	
	Rt	Lt	Rt	Lt	Rt	Lt	Rt	Lt
Number of active ulcers	None		1		2		≥3	
	Rt	Lt	Rt	Lt	Rt	Lt	Rt	Lt
Active ulcer duration (longest active)	None		<3 mo		>3 mo, <1 y		>1 y	
	Rt	Lt	Rt	Lt	Rt	Lt	Rt	Lt
Active ulcer size (largest active)	None		<2 cm		2–6 cm		>6 cm	
	Rt	Lt	Rt	Lt	Rt	Lt	Rt	Lt
Compression therapy	Not used		Intermittent		Most days		Daily	
	Rt	Lt	Rt	Lt	Rt	Lt	Rt	Lt

VCSS – RIGHT: _____ VCSS – LEFT: _____

Abbreviations: Lt, left; Rt, right; VCSS-R, Venous Clinical Severity Score–Right.
Source: *Seminars in Interventional Radiology Vol. 38 No. 2/2021.*

8.2 Indications/Contraindications for Recanalization in CTO

Some experts suggest treatment of central CTO based on the severity of symptoms on presentation and not the venographic findings. There are some patients with extensive occlusions that may be asymptomatic or mildly symptomatic and do not warrant treatment in our opinion. Indications for treatment include patients with significant limb symptoms such as pain, swelling, venous dermatitis, ulcers, and recurrent cellulitis, which

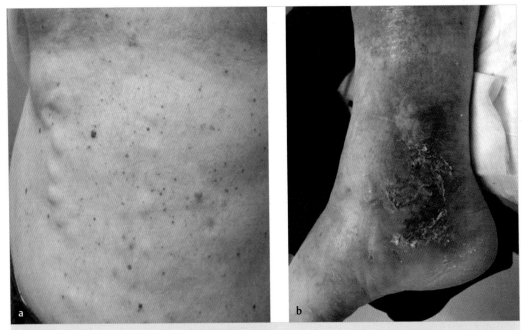

Fig. 8.1 (a) Extensive collateral formation in the abdomen from a patient with central chronic total occlusion (CTO). **(b)** Venous ulcer. Note hemosiderosis, classic location at medial malleolus, crusting, edema, and shallow irregular borders. Source: *Seminars in Interventional Radiology 2018; 35(05): 399-405.*

should be elucidated from a thorough history and physical examination. Symptomatic patients who have failed conservative therapy with AC and compression stockings should also be treated. Most institutes also use the CEAP clinical stage ≥ 3 to accept patients for endovascular treatment for central CTO recanalization.

Patients who have had recent major surgery, prior recent cerebrovascular hemorrhage, recent cardiopulmonary resuscitation (CPR), pregnant patients, or those with severe coagulopathy should not be considered as candidates for central CTO revascularization. Special considerations such as phlegmasia cerulea dolens from CTO may benefit from surgical thrombectomy rather than recanalization if there is profound limb ischemia with muscle weakness and sensory loss.[21] This is generally because of the acute nature of the pathology and the need for emergent intervention. Other exclusion criteria generally used are life expectancy < 5 years, severe chronic obstructive pulmonary disease (COPD), cardiac failure, and malignant disease due to the risk/benefit ratio of the procedure in these settings.

8.3 Patient Selection and Preprocedure Workup

Clinical judgment should be used on a case-by-case basis to decide on interventional therapy. Timing of DVT, associated risk factors for the development of DVT, prolonged anesthesia, contraindications to postoperative AC, age, and prognosis of the patient all need to be considered. Lower extremity recanalization patients can often tolerate sedation; however, with iliocaval recanalization, general anesthesia may be used. Therefore, risk factors associated with prolonged anesthesia need to be considered. If bilateral CTO of the iliac veins are present, a suggested strategy is to evaluate each limb separately during the workup. A good strategy to guide patient selection is to evaluate and grade venous claudication with walking various distances (e.g., < 50, < 200, and > 200 m). This can be done in the outpatient setting with the use of a treadmill exercise challenge test, and the distance at which the claudication becomes severe enough to discontinue the exercise should be recorded.[22]

As with any intervention, imaging is needed to determine the location and extent of the affected vessels prior to attempting recanalization in central CTOs. Ultrasound evaluation of the lower extremity is sufficient prior to intervention; however, the central venous system is more accurately assessed with computed tomography (CT) venography, magnetic resonance (MR) venogram, or angiography to determine the extent and location of the clot. Ultrasound offers the advantage of being a noninvasive, cheap, and easily repeatable study. Criteria for establishing a significant central venous stenosis in the iliocaval system have been documented. Duplex ultrasound (DU) showing a V2/V1 gradient > 2.5 has been shown to correlate with symptom severity and should be used as a guideline directing intervention.[23] This value detected 90% of significant stenosis when compared to venography and intravascular ultrasound (IVUS). Similar values have been reported in the literature for determining significant stenosis in dialysis access and portal venous system. A V2/V1 ratio > 3.0 has been used for detecting significant stenosis in portosystemic stents and the anastomosis of dialysis access, and V2/V1 > 2.0 for the vein proximal to the anastomosis.[24,25] We also suggest DU of the lower extremity and pelvis prior to recanalization for detection of superficial and/or deep reflux and collateral pathways. Stenosis that has significant asymmetric flow in the common femoral vein (CFV) and the presence of collateral pathways (e.g., flow reversal in the internal iliac vein) are considered significant if there is a > 50% stenosis of the vessel lumen.

8.4 Technique

The technique for approaching recanalization in central CTOs differs from CDT and mechanical thrombectomy. The goal is to cross a chronic venous occlusion, and special consideration needs to be given to collateral venous pathways, guidewire course, patient positioning, and access site.

8.4.1 Equipment

Catheter and mechanical thrombolysis will be addressed briefly in this section as they do play a part in recanalization of CTO once the stenotic segment is crossed. Mechanical thrombectomy equipment falls into two major categories: rotation and rheolytic devices. Rotational devices such as the Trerotola Percutaneous Thrombectomy Device (Arrow International, Reading, PA) have a high-velocity rotating helix cage made of nitinol attached to a drive cable to macerate clot.[26] There are centers with significant experience with this device in treating CTO of dialysis grafts with expectations for a larger version device aimed at treating central CTOs available in the near future. Rheolytic devices such as AngioJet (Boston Scientific, Maple Grove, MN) utilize high-pressure saline jets to fragment thrombus. The device creates a negative pressure zone that draws the thrombus toward the catheter where it is aspirated and removed. Case reports of hemolysis, bradycardia, or hemoglobinuria have been reported while using this device and so device running time must be taken into consideration especially during lengthy procedures.[27,28] Ultrasound devices such as the EKOS catheter (EKOS Corporation, Bothwell, WA) contain multiple ultrasound transducers that radially emit high-frequency, low-energy ultrasound. It is thought that the ultrasound exposes plasminogen receptor sites on the surface of the clot by expanding and thinning the fibrin. The ultrasound then forces thrombolytic into the clot where it stays and dissolves the clot over time.[29] Some authors advocate using AngioJet for acute (< 28 days) clot and EKOS thrombolysis for chronic DVT. Garcia recently published a treatment algorithm for CTOs including chronic clot extending into the iliac veins and IVC.[30] Once the diseased venous segment is crossed, serial venoplasty of each involved segment up to the size of the corresponding normal patient vein is performed. After dilation, stenting is performed to the level of the inguinal ligament. EKOS catheters are left overnight at an infusion rate of 0.5 mg/h our with pneumatic compression boots overnight. The following day, additional venography and further interventions including venoplasty and stenting are performed if needed. There are no patency data available using this technique for central CTOs and, therefore, it is mentioned here for completeness.

8.4.2 Patient Positioning/Access/Technique

The authors perform procedures starting with the patient in the prone position with the flexibility to reposition at any time during the procedure. Lovenox has become the authors' AC of choice due to its more constant anticoagulant effect than heparin, anti-inflammatory effects, and lack of partial thromboplastin time (PTT) monitoring needed as with heparin. Initial access site at our institution is below the level of occlusion, often from the posterior tibial vein or other deep vein. If the entire below- and above-knee popliteal vein is patent, then the popliteal vein is accessed. After the vein is punctured under ultrasound guidance, a vascular sheath is inserted and a diagnostic venogram is performed to visualize the extent of the thrombosis. Initial attempt at crossing the occlusion may be performed using either a multipurpose catheter or angled-tip catheter with a hydrophilic road runner guidewire supported by a ridged braided sheath. The wire tip can be looped to find the correct course and prevent entry into parallel channels. If it is unable to cross the lesion, the road runner can be exchanged for a stiff glidewire to cross the occlusion. If it is still unsuccessful in crossing the lesion, the authors suggest using an additional access site to cross from both ends of the occlusion until "through-and-through" wire access is established. This can be done by snaring the wire from an additional access site such as the right internal jugular vein and allows for better

stability for stenting (▶ Fig. 8.2). Entry into the IVC is characterized by easy advancement of the wire into the right atrium at approximately the level of the 9th or 10th rib.

At this point, if there is still an inability to cross the lesion, there are additional techniques to consider. Tunneling devices such as the Frontrunner CTO (Cordis) and the PowerWire Radiofrequency (RF) guidewire (Baylis Medical Company Inc, Montreal, QC) have been promoted for recanalizing the most stubborn, chronic central venous occlusions. The Frontrunner XP CTO is a blunt dissecting catheter that was designed to bore through fibrotic vascular occlusions. The majority of its use has been for arterial occlusions; however, anecdotal case reports have been published using these devices in CTOs.[31] Additionally, the RF thermal wire has been used successfully to cross lesions that cannot be recanalized using conventional techniques.[32] The PowerWire has been cleared by the Food and Drug Administration (FDA) for use in facilitating crossing chronically occluded blood vessels. It is a 0.035-inch low-friction guidewire that deliveries RF energy at its tip when connected

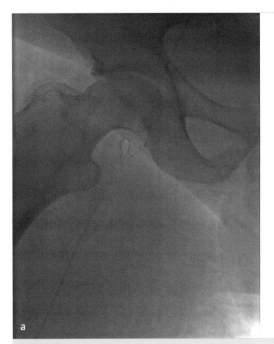
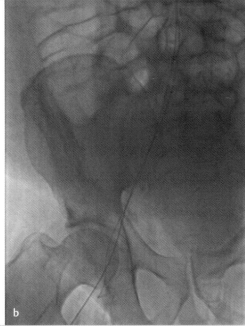

Fig. 8.2 (a) Through-and-through access prior to stenting in a previously completely occluded right chronic venous insufficiency (CIV). Access was via the popliteal and right internal jugular (IJ) vein in this case. **(b)** A 10-mm gooseneck snare was used to grab the wire from the jugular approach and pull it thought the neck.

to a power supply. The cost of the wire is approximately $875 per case and there are three different tips available (straight, 45-degree angled, relaxed 45 degrees). Successful recanalization using the RF wire has been reported in 42 patients in the upper venous system.[33] Other authors have described using this device successfully in the management of hemodialysis occlusions as well as lower extremity deep veins.[34,35] We have no experience with this technique, but it has proven to be a useful adjuvant to have in the Interventional Radiologist (IR) toolbox when dealing with complex CTOs.

A final technique worth examining, and the most commonly used by the authors, is the sharp recanalization technique used to recanalize chronic central venous occlusions. The majority of cases using this technique have been reported in the upper venous system to place central venous catheters (CVCs) in patients who have run out of access as well as to alleviate the symptoms of SVC occlusion. This technique attempts to create through-and-through access from a femoral and upper arm access site with the use of a gooseneck snare as a target for puncture in the neck area for placement of CVCs.[36] Once the needle is correctly placed at the center of the snare, a 0.018-inch guidewire is then advanced through the snare. The tract is then dilated and an Amplatz stiff-type exchange guidewire is advanced through the micropuncture set dilator and retrieved with the snare through the femoral access site. This through-and-through access can then allow subsequent balloon dilation and catheter placement. Recent case series reported by Arabi et al demonstrates a series of seven patients who all had successful central CTO recanalization using this technique.[37] Through-and-through access was obtained via a right upper arm and femoral vein access site using a 10-mm Amplatz gooseneck snare as a target by puncturing the right brachiocephalic vein.

Some authors have described starting with the internal jugular vein to establish retrograde catheterization of the main CFV.[38] With occlusions in the iliocaval system, the authors find the length of the catheters and pushability is superior from a popliteal approach or depending on the inferior extent of the occlusion, a greater saphenous vein approach. Recanalization rates are also much lower when there is an occluded common iliac veins and IVC via the retrograde approach.[39] Midthigh access has also been described as an initial access site approach.[40] Studies have shown similar

recanalization rates with this approach and demonstrate that the more proximal the access site for iliocaval recanalization, the more likely an adequate landing zone for stent placement will be achieved.

It is worthwhile to note that during this portion of the procedure, perforations of the venous system are common and are not a cause to abort. If the recanalization is unsuccessful, the perforated vein will not have sustained flow. If the recanalization is successful, then the venous return to the heart will follow the path of least resistance (i.e., the newly patent stent) and venous pressures will become negligible and the perforation will seal by itself (▶ Fig. 8.3).

8.4.3 Balloon Angioplasty/Stenting

Stenting is the initial procedure of choice once central CTOs have been recanalized. The objective is to restore flow through the main central venous system (common femoral, iliac, and caval) and outcompete collateral vessel flow.[41] Angioplasty and stenting in the setting of obstruction is well documented at improving the quality of lives of patients with symptomatic CTOs.[42] Prior to stenting, the authors recommend predilatation of all stenotic segments with balloon angioplasty using large (16- to 24-mm) noncompliant balloons to high pressures (20 atm). The use of high-pressure noncompliant balloons will allow any perivenous fibrotic tissue outside the vein to be broken as well as disrupting any intraluminal venous scarring.

Thought should be given to the choice of stent configuration, length, diameter, and position in order to achieve optimum clinical outcomes. Self-expanding metallic stents historically have had good results on venous lesions. Balloon expandable stents originally showed promising immediate results in the venous system; however, iterative thrombosis rates increase compared to self-expanding stents after 2 months of intervention.[43] Optimal stent diameters in the common femoral, iliac, and caval systems in most patients range from 12 to 14, 12 to 16, and 16 to 24 mm, respectively. In order to determine stent length, the authors advocate using IVUS routinely.[44] This technique has shown superior results when assessing stenoses, stent diameter, and stent placement versus single-plane venography.

In stenting central CTOs, stents may be placed throughout most of the entirety of the central venous system. Stents have been deployed across the

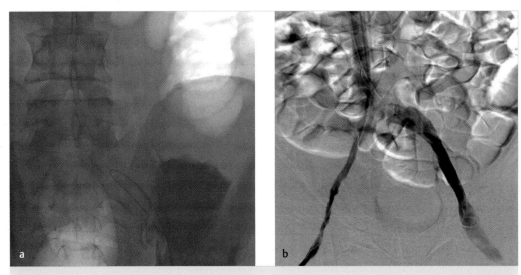

Fig. 8.3 (a) Perforation of the left common iliac vein during an iliocaval recanalization. **(b)** One day later, the perforation sealed off and was not evident on venography.

renal or hepatic vein entry into the IVC without adverse effects.[45] The proximal extent of the stent should be no further than the level of the atrium, but not into the atrium. Extensive investigation has been done to determine the role of stenting across the inguinal ligament and data are controversial. Neglén et al published that, contrary to stenting in the arterial system, in which stenting across the inguinal ligament is contraindicated, in the venous system it can be done safely with braided, stainless steel stents.[46] They showed no increase in-stent fracture, narrowing due to external compression, development of focal severe in-stent stenosis, and no effect on long-term patency in stents placed across the ligament. They conclude that patency rates are dependent on the etiology of the CTO and whether the treated obstruction is occlusive or nonocclusive. This is due to occlusive obstructions having lower secondary patency rates overall. A recent study by Ye et al addressed this issue as well, and concluded that long stents extending below the inguinal ligament had a higher rate of in-stent restenosis in the first 12 months.[47] They included the presence of visible collaterals after the procedure as also having a higher rate of in-stent restenosis and did not give specific mention to the contribution of this group to the inguinal ligament group. The length of the stents was also the only variable that was associated with in-stent restenosis that was statistically significant ($p < 0.5$).

Further research needs to be done in this area. It is the authors' opinion that stents can be placed across the inguinal ligament if all attempts at gaining flow from the femoral vein into the CFV and iliac veins are unsuccessful. The authors do not recommend placement of stents below the level of the lesser trochanter and/or within the femoral or popliteal veins. At the end of the procedure, venography is performed to examine the sheath, to evaluate for residual thromboembolic complications or stenosis, and to exclude stent recoil.

8.5 Postprocedural Management

All sites are compressed with bandages without using a closure device even when large sheaths are used (up to 10 Fr). Following recanalization, 20 to 30 mm Hg thigh-high stockings should be placed on the patient. For iliocaval recanalization, which the authors do under general anesthesia, patients are admitted to the hospital for 2 to 4 days. It is not uncommon for patients to have back pain from stenting and laying on the table, nausea from anesthesia, and significant fatigue after undergoing a 6- to 8-hour procedure. Routine iliofemoral CTO recanalization is done under moderate sedation with the patient leaving the same or next day.

Venous recanalization causes significant disruption of the venous endothelium and patients are in a hypercoagulable state for a few weeks, which

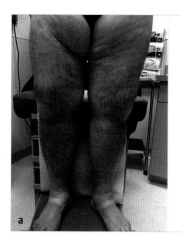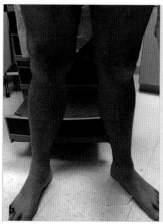

Fig. 8.4 **(a)** A 44-year-old man with > 3 years of chronic lower extremity swelling and pain with complete iliocaval chronic total occlusion (CTO). **(b)** One month after recanalization and stenting his IVC and iliac veins and symptom free (right).

necessitates optimum intraprocedural and postprocedural AC. The interventionalist will often be required to manage the medication in an outpatient setting. If a patient prior to the procedure was on indefinite AC, he or she will likely continue to require indefinite treatment. For patients who had a remote DVT in the past requiring AC treatment and have since been off AC, we recommend low-molecular-weight heparin (LMWH) 1 mg/kg twice a day starting 2 days prior to the procedure and for 1 month postprocedure followed by a newer novel anticoagulant for 6 months. For those with a history of heparin-induced thrombocytopenia (HIT) or an allergy to heparin, argatroban is used during the case and fondaparinux is used postprocedure. If injections are not tolerated, warfarin can be used and started the same day as the procedure with a target international normalized ratio (INR) of 2 to 3. A heparin or LMWH bridge should be used until consecutive INRs are therapeutic.[48] The duration of therapy is a topic of debate, and it should be up to the interventionalist to address at a follow-up visit. At the 6-month visit, the risk of recurrent in-stent thrombosis should be determined based on the patient's symptoms and imaging findings and weighed against the risk of bleeding. We also advocate using a concomitant antiplatelet agent such clopidogrel (Plavix) and/or aspirin for 1 month. Recent data suggest that concomitant antiplatelet therapy is associated with reduced stent malfunction following iliocaval stenting (hazard ratio of 0.28); however, this protocol is institution dependent and the evidence is largely extrapolated from arterial studies.[49]

Patient follow-up visits should be scheduled at 1, 6, and 12 months and then annually. On follow-up visit, we suggest analyzing pain on a scale from 0 to 10 and swelling on a grade scale from 0 to 2. Grade 0 is no swelling, grade 1 is visible ankle edema, and grade 2 is edema encompassing the entire leg. The Chronic Venous Insufficiency Questionnaire (CIVIQ) is a good tool that has been used to assess quality-of-life metrics.[50] VCSS and CEAP scores as mentioned earlier should be calculated at each follow-up visit. Documenting resolution of symptoms cosmetically with digital photography is also a useful tool to track patient progress (▶ Fig. 8.4).

DU is an effective method to follow up venous intervention results at follow-up examinations. This method has been shown to be sensitive in identifying clinically significant venous stenosis after recanalization and stent placement. Preliminary results show that it is comparable to venography in assessing stent patency.[23] Peak vein velocity gradients of > 2.5 across the stenosis is the best accepted diagnostic criteria to assesses for restenosis; however, thrombosis and reflux can also be detected. Other authors routinely perform contrast venography at 6 to 12 weeks after intervention.[51] Although the authors advocate follow-up initially with ultrasound if the patient's body habitus permits, CT venography is commonly performed to assess stent patency and restenosis.

8.6 Complications/Special Considerations

Complications associated with central CTO recanalization are of two types, and both will be addressed here. There are complications related to the procedure itself and those related to the inciting cause of the CTO in the first place. The most common postoperative complication encountered by us and other authors is back pain. Ye et al reported approximately 50% of patients undergoing stent placement for postthrombotic CTO had back pain after the procedure.[47] In our opinion, postprocedure back pain is not an urgent cause for alarm and usually resolves and can be managed conservatively with over-the-counter (OTC) analgesics or prescription narcotics if pain is severe. Other encountered procedural complications include guidewires being caught in stents, postoperative swelling, and stent thrombosis. As mentioned earlier, perforation is an unavoidable complication that should not be a cause to abort the procedure. There have been case reports of retroperitoneal bleeding from high cannulation sites requiring transfusion as well as arterial injuries requiring open repair.[45] It should be noted that all these occurred before the use of ultrasound guidance.

8.6.1 CTO due to IVC Filter Occlusion

IVC filter occlusion is a common cause of central CTOs. This is largely due to the interventionalist placing these filters, sometimes, under soft indications and not following up to ensure they were removed. Some degree of IVC thrombosis rates on follow-up examination by CT has been report as high

as 18.6%. The vast majority of patients are asymptomatic, and total occlusion of the filter-bearing IVC was seen only in 2% of the patients.[52,53] However, in this population of patients, this can be severely debilitating and recanalization should be addressed.[54] For filter occlusions, we recommend removal of the filter if the interventionalist has experience with complex filter retrieval prior to recanalization. Filter retrieval has technical success rates as high as 97% with no difference in patency rates between retrieved and excluded filters.[55,56] Alternatively, using an angioplasty balloon to crush and displace the filter laterally is a favored technique because it pushes the filter away from the aorta and duodenum, which are more medial to the IVC. We describe here the case of a 62-year-old man status post coronary artery bypass graft (CABG) and aortic valve replacement (AVR) 3 days prior to our facility with IVC thrombosis approximately 3 weeks after his filter was placed. It was determined that he was not a candidate for thrombolysis and he was discharged home on Lovenox. He underwent DVT lysis 6 weeks later at our facility (▶ Fig. 8.5).

8.6.2 Stent Migration/ Malpositioning

Special consideration needs to be given to complications related to stenting given that stenting is the gold standard for recanalization of iliofemoral and iliocaval CTOs. Misplaced and inappropriately

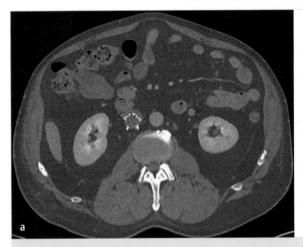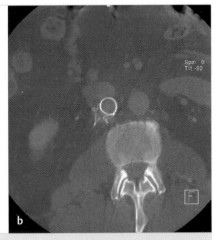

Fig. 8.5 (a) Computed tomography (CT venogram on presentation showing complete occlusion of the inferior vena cava (IVC) and and IVC filter present. **(b)** Dyna-CT post recanalization and stent placement. Note the location of the filter relative to the stent.

sized stents increase the likelihood of stent migration and other complications. For migrated stents in the face of chronic occlusion, we recommend attempted retrieval as the stent may serve as a possible source of embolus to the heart and pulmonary vasculature. This is especially true if the occlusion is occurring distal to the stent and the proximal end is free floating. We describe here the case of a 43-year-old obese man with a history of congenital lymphedema and venous insufficiency who presented to the emergency department with severe pain of the right lower extremity (RLE). Three weeks prior to presentation, the patient underwent failed thrombolytic therapy for an RLE DVT performed by a vascular surgeon at an outside hospital. Initial examination of the RLE revealed exquisite pain upon palpation and diffuse, nonpitting edema to the level of the midthigh. CT angiography revealed a nonocclusive thrombus in the right external iliac vein and occlusive thrombosis extending from the right CFV to the popliteal vein. Additionally, an intravascular stent at the junction between the IVC and the right common iliac vein was identified, which exhibited minimal apposition to the vessel wall (▶ Fig. 8.6).

Access to the stent was obtained after overnight CDT and AngioJet therapy to recanalize the chronic occlusion in the right CFV extending to the popliteal vein. The maldeployed 10-mm Zilver Cook stent was noticed to have been free on all surfaces in the proximal portion of the IVC. It was decided to use a monorail approach with two 25-mm gooseneck snare catheters to retrieve the stent. The first snare was attached to the midportion of the stent (▶ Fig. 8.7a) and the second snare was attached to the proximal portion of the stent

(▶ Fig. 8.7b). The snares were then closed and the stent was oversheathed and retrieved from the jugular access (▶ Fig. 8.7c).

8.6.3 Stents Trapped in Filters

Another interesting problem that may be encountered during recanalization for central CTOs is migration of stents that become lodged within IVC filters. The case below is a 44-year-old man who presented to our facility with extensive lower extremity DVT, pain, and swelling. He was unable to walk long distances, wear shoes, or wear compression stockings on presentation. His past medical history was significant for having bilateral pulmonary embolus necessitating IVC filter placement 3 years prior to presentation at our facility. Previously, he had also undergone stenting of the right common iliac vein (CIV) for chronic RLE edema. CT venography demonstrated chronic occlusive thrombus in his iliocaval system and the previously placed right iliac vein stent that had migrated and become trapped within the filter. IVC and bilateral iliac vein recanalization with an attempt at filter/stent removal was attempted (▶ Fig. 8.8).

From a right internal jugular vein approach, the authors attempted to oversheath the entire filter/stent complex. This was unsuccessful as the struts of the stent prevented the filter from being oversheathed (▶ Fig. 8.9). A snare was then used to grab the inferior portion of the stent and simultaneously pull down on the stent and oversheath the filter. Careful consideration was then given to the stent, which was now a free foreign body within the IVC. While the stent was still attached to the snare, we placed a 24 mm × 70 mm Wallstent in

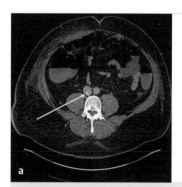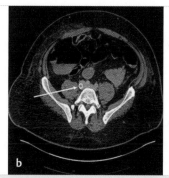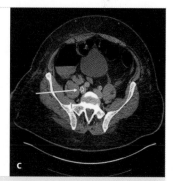

Fig. 8.6 Computed tomography (CT) venogram demonstrating a 10-mm Zilver Cook stent within the **(a)** inferior vena cava (IVC) extending **(b)** caudally and **(c)** at the iliocaval confluence.

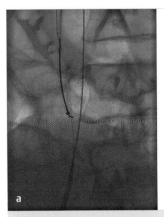 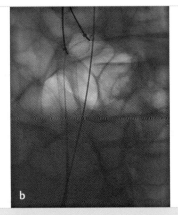 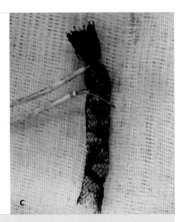

Fig. 8.7 Retrieval of a vascular stent during central chronic total occlusion (CTO) recanalization. **(a)** Through-and-through access was obtained and the free proximal portion of the stent was snared. **(b)** Monorail approach ensured adequate purchase on the stent. **(c)** Postretrieval stent.

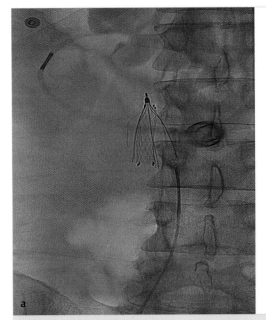 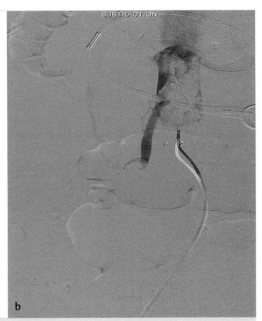

Fig. 8.8 (a) Initial fluoroscopic images after recanalization of the iliacs demonstrating a stent present within an inferior vena cava (IVC) filter. **(b)** Postcontrast images showing near-complete occlusion of the IVC filter with reflux down a collateral pathway adjacent to the IVC.

the IVC crushing the indwelling stent against the caval wall (▶ Fig. 8.10).

There have been several studies looking at percutaneous foreign body retrievals, but few that include misplaced stents especially during central

CTO recanalization. Most case reports of stent misplacement and retrieval occur immediately after the stent has been deployed.[57,58] The rate of stent migration/misplacement has been reported to occur in up to 3% of cases and while most of these

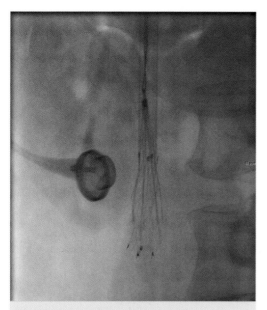

Fig. 8.9 Stent strut preventing oversheathing of the entire filter/stent complex.

are recognized immediately, a small percentage are found on subsequent follow-up.[59] It is important to recognize these events early and attempt retrieval of the misplaced stent due to the vascular complications that could occur, leading to more difficult recanalization as well as iliofemoral/iliocaval thrombosis. Other serious complications due to vascular stent migration include pulmonary infarctions following migration into the pulmonary arteries or myocardial injury as a result of stents migrating into the right ventricle.[60]

A case series was published by Gabelmann et al looking at percutaneous retrieval techniques used for 28 patients with maldeployed or migrated endovascular stents.[61] The retrieval methods used in these patients included balloon catheters, gooseneck snares, grasping forceps, as well as the placement of additional stents to effectively oppose the misplaced stent to the vessel wall. Twenty-six of the 28 cases were recognized immediately and retrieved. The two stents not recognized immediately were transjugular intrahepatic portosystemic shunt (TIPS) stents discovered after 2 and 10 days

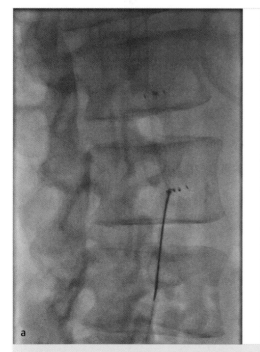

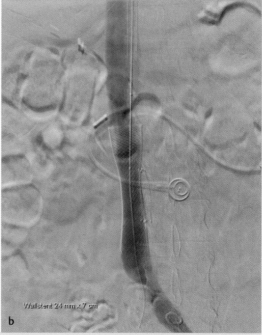

Fig. 8.10 (a) Snare attached to the free-floating stent in the inferior vena cava (IVC). **(b)** A 24 mm × 7 cm Wallstent placed in the IVC crushing the stent against the caval wall.

and no percutaneous retrieval techniques were attempted. These stents remained in the pulmonary artery of the left lobe of the lung and were followed over a mean of 42 months with no adverse consequences. It is the authors' opinion that if a stent/filter can be retrieved easily, it should be done. However, if there are risk factors that put the patient at an unacceptable risk, it should be either crushed or left in place provided the patient is not symptomatic.

8.7 Clinical Data and Outcomes

We included in our summary of clinical outcomes large studies of > 30 patients with follow-up durations > 2 years after recanalization for thrombotic central CTOs in the iliocaval and iliofemoral segments (▶ Table 8.3).

The majority of the lesions in these studies were documented as older than 6 months on recanalization and all patients met a CEAP criteria of at least C ≥ 3. Technical success is defined here as restoration of venous flow on final venogram after recanalization and stent placement. This included if there was reduction in blood flow or collateralization on initial venogram. Technical success rates for all studies analyzed were high (83–95%). Patency rates are the major determining factors when it comes to clinical success and reinterventions, and understanding their definitions is important in reporting clinical outcomes. Primary patency is defined as < 50% restenosis on follow-up without any reinterventions. Primary assisted patency is confirmed patency on

follow-up after reintervention (e.g., angioplasty) to maintain patency. Finally, secondary patency is defined as reestablishment of flow with angioplasty, thrombolysis, or stent placement after reocclusion of the previously treated vein segments. A major distinction is made in primary patency rates between nonthrombotic and postthrombotic limb recanalization. One of the largest studies to date by Neglén et al in 2007 looked at 982 limbs for obstructive iliac vein lesions that were treated by stenting.[65] Only 6% of these had iliac veins that required recanalization. In this group, the occlusion rate was much higher than that of nonocclusive iliac vein stenosis (24 vs. 3%). The focus of this chapter is specifically on central CTO recanalization; therefore, nonocclusive stenosis was not included in this review.

Clinical success is defined as significant reduction of symptoms during the duration of follow-up of the studies. These include reduction in pain and swelling, resolution of venous ulcers, and quality-of-life metrics. A good metric, as stated before, to monitor clinical process is by using a venous-specific quality-of-life questionnaire combined with the Villalta score. Of the studies included, only Ye et al used the Villalta scoring system and comparison of quality-of-life metrics is difficult without a standardized reporting format (▶ Table 8.4). An important finding from these studies is that limbs of patients who had bilateral stenting had a higher frequency of reocclusion (57 vs. 27%). Other factors associated with stent occlusions included prior thrombosis, male sex, recent trauma, and age < 50 years.

Table 8.3 Clinical outcomes from recanalization in central CTOs

Study	Treated limbs	Clinical outcomes
Kölbel et al[62]	57	75% overall improvement in symptoms (limb swelling and pain combined)
Raju and Neglén[40]	139	Pain and swelling improvement in 79 and 66%, ulceration healing in 56%, and improvement in all quality-of-life metrics by CVIQ
Rosales et al[63]	32	Pain and swelling improvement in 94% (combined), ulceration healing in 57%, VCSS in C3/C6 patients 9 (5–12) and 21 (18–29) pre-op and 1 (0–11) and 7 (6–14) post-op
Ye et al[47]	112	Pain and swelling improvement 72 and 70%, ulceration healing in 78% (36/46), total Villalta PTS score 22 pre-op and 9.3 post-op
Murphy et al[64]	60	Pain and swelling improvement in 91 and 83%, ulceration healing in 78%, VCSS 8.4 ± 5.1 pre-op and 3.9 ± 3.2 post-op

Abbreviations: CTO, chronic total occlusion; PTS, postthrombotic syndrome; VCSS, Venous Clinical Severity Score.

Table 8.4 The Villalta scale

Symptoms scored by the patient	Signs scored by caregiver (nurse/physician)
Pain	Pretibial edema
Cramps	Skin induration
Heaviness	Hyperpigmentation
Paresthesia	Redness
Itching	Venous ectasia
	Pain on calf compression

Ulcer is scored as present or absent

Note: All symptoms and signs are scored from 0 (absent) to 3 (severe) and summarized to produce a total score ranging from 0 to 33. A total score of ≥5 points corresponds to any grade of postthrombotic syndrome (PTS), 5 to 14 points to mild/moderate PTS, and ≥15 points or the presence of a venous ulcer to severe PTS. A score of less than 5 indicates no PTS.
Source: *Semin Thromb Hemost 2017; 43(05): 500-504.*

The Acute Venous Thrombosis: Thrombus Removal with Adjunctive Catheter-Directed Thrombolysis (ATTRACT) trial compared pharmacomechanical CDT (PCDT) to AC alone, measuring the VCSS and the Villalta PTS score as outcomes at up to 2 years' follow-up. While there was no significant difference in the development of PTS between groups, the severity of symptoms as determined by mean VCSS and Villalta scores was significantly lower in the PCDT group at all follow-up visits ($p \leq 0.01$) except for the VCSS scores at 24 months ($p = 0.03$). PCDT was associated with a significantly higher major bleed risk of 1.7% compared to 0.3% on AC alone; however, no patients in either arm suffered intracranial bleeds.[62]

A recent subgroup analysis of ATTRACT patients with acute iliofemoral DVT demonstrated that PCDT had a greater reduction in acute pain and swelling symptoms ($p < 0.01$) and increased venous disease-specific quality of life as measured by VEINES-QOL scores ($p = 0.029$). There was no significant difference in bleed risk or recurrent VTE.[63] The findings of the ATTRACT trial and its subgroup analysis suggest that PCDT is an effective method to reduce symptom severity and improve quality of life in patients with acute iliofemoral DVT.

8.8 Conclusion

Recanalization of central chronic venous occlusions (CTOs) is a technique that has been gaining increasing popularity over the past 10 to 15 years with the advancements in endovascular techniques. Therefore, proper understanding of the tools and techniques used by interventional radiologist to set up a successful practice that includes DVT interventions is essential. Quality of life can be significantly improved in patients who suffer with PTS if they are managed appropriately from initial intervention using the strategies described in this chapter.

References

[1] O'Dea J, Schainfeld RM. Venous interventions. Circ Cardiovasc Interv. 2014; 7(2):256–265

[2] Heit JA. The epidemiology of venous thromboembolism in the community. Arterioscler Thromb Vasc Biol. 2008; 28(3): 370–372

[3] Hippisley-Cox J, Coupland C. Development and validation of risk prediction algorithm (QThrombosis) to estimate future risk of venous thromboembolism: prospective cohort study. BMJ. 2011; 343:d4656

[4] Knipp BS, Ferguson E, Williams DM, et al. Factors associated with outcome after interventional treatment of symptomatic iliac vein compression syndrome. J Vasc Surg. 2007; 46(4): 743–749

[5] Neglén P. Chronic venous obstruction: diagnostic considerations and therapeutic role of percutaneous iliac stenting. Vascular. 2007; 15(5):273–280

[6] Vedantham S, Thorpe PE, Cardella JF, et al. CIRSE and SIR Standards of Practice Committees. Quality improvement guidelines for the treatment of lower extremity deep vein thrombosis with use of endovascular thrombus removal. J Vasc Interv Radiol. 2009; 20(7) Suppl:S227–S239

[7] Akesson H, Brudin L, Dahlström JA, Eklöf B, Ohlin P, Plate G. Venous function assessed during a 5 year period after acute ilio-femoral venous thrombosis treated with anticoagulation. Eur J Vasc Surg. 1990; 4(1):43–48

[8] Raju S. Treatment of iliac-caval outflow obstruction. Semin Vasc Surg. 2015; 28(1):47–53

[9] Eklöf B, Rutherford RB, Bergan JJ, et al. American Venous Forum International Ad Hoc Committee for Revision of the CEAP Classification. Revision of the CEAP classification for chronic venous disorders: consensus statement. J Vasc Surg. 2004; 40(6):1248–1252

[10] Gloviczki P, Comerota AJ, Dalsing MC, et al. Society for Vascular Surgery, American Venous Forum. The care of patients with varicose veins and associated chronic venous diseases: clinical practice guidelines of the Society for Vascular Surgery and the American Venous Forum. J Vasc Surg. 2011; 53(5) Suppl:2S–48S

[11] Vasquez MA, Rabe E, McLafferty RB, et al. American Venous Forum Ad Hoc Outcomes Working Group. Revision of the Venous Clinical Severity Score: venous outcomes consensus statement: special communication of the American Venous Forum Ad Hoc Outcomes Working Group. J Vasc Surg. 2010; 52(5):1387–1396

[12] Rutherford RB, Padberg FT, Jr, Comerota AJ, Kistner RL, Meissner MH, Moneta GL. Venous severity scoring: an adjunct to venous outcome assessment. J Vasc Surg. 2000; 31(6):1307–1312

[13] Pesavento R, Bernardi E, Concolato A, Dalla Valle F, Pagnan A, Prandoni P. Postthrombotic syndrome. Semin Thromb Hemost. 2006; 32(7):744–751

[14] Prandoni P, Kahn SR. Post-thrombotic syndrome: prevalence, prognostication and need for progress. Br J Haematol. 2009; 145(3):286–295

[15] Prandoni P, Lensing AW, Cogo A, et al. The long-term clinical course of acute deep venous thrombosis. Ann Intern Med. 1996; 125(1):1–7

[16] Lindner DJ, Edwards JM, Phinney ES, Taylor LM, Jr, Porter JM. Long-term hemodynamic and clinical sequelae of lower extremity deep vein thrombosis. J Vasc Surg. 1986; 4(5):436–442

[17] Sharafuddin MJ, Sun S, Hoballah JJ, Youness FM, Sharp WJ, Roh BS. Endovascular management of venous thrombotic and occlusive diseases of the lower extremities. J Vasc Interv Radiol. 2003; 14(4):405–423

[18] Plate G, Eklöf B, Norgren L, Ohlin P, Dahlström JA. Venous thrombectomy for iliofemoral vein thrombosis: 10-year results of a prospective randomised study. Eur J Vasc Endovasc Surg. 1997; 14(5):367–374

[19] Soosainathan A, Moore HM, Gohel MS, Davies AH. Scoring systems for the post-thrombotic syndrome. J Vasc Surg. 2013; 57(1):254–261

[20] Kahn SR, Partsch H, Vedantham S, Prandoni P, Kearon C, Subcommittee on Control of Anticoagulation of the Scientific and Standardization Committee of the International Society on Thrombosis and Haemostasis. Definition of post-thrombotic syndrome of the leg for use in clinical investigations: a recommendation for standardization. J Thromb Haemost. 2009; 7(5):879–883

[21] Yang SS, Yun WS. Surgical thrombectomy for phlegmasia cerulea dolens. Vasc Spec Int. 2016; 32(4):201–204

[22] Delis KT, Bountouroglou D, Mansfield AO. Venous claudication in iliofemoral thrombosis: long-term effects on venous hemodynamics, clinical status, and quality of life. Ann Surg. 2004; 239(1):118–126

[23] Labropoulos N, Borge M, Pierce K, Pappas PJ. Criteria for defining significant central vein stenosis with duplex ultrasound. J Vasc Surg. 2007; 46(1):101–107

[24] Grogan J, Castilla M, Lozanski L, Griffin A, Loth F, Bassiouny H. Frequency of critical stenosis in primary arteriovenous fistulae before hemodialysis access: should duplex ultrasound surveillance be the standard of care? J Vasc Surg. 2005; 41(6):1000–1006

[25] Crossin JD, Muradali D, Wilson SR. US of liver transplants: normal and abnormal. Radiographics. 2003; 23(5):1093–1114

[26] Trerotola SO, Vesely TM, Lund GB, Soulen MC, Ehrman KO, Cardella JF, Arrow-Trerotola Percutaneous Thrombolytic Device Clinical Trial. Treatment of thrombosed hemodialysis access grafts: Arrow-Trerotola percutaneous thrombolytic device versus pulse-spray thrombolysis. Radiology. 1998; 206(2):403–414

[27] Jeyabalan G, Saba S, Baril DT, Makaroun MS, Chaer RA. Bradyarrhythmias during rheolytic pharmacomechanical thrombectomy for deep vein thrombosis. J Endovasc Ther. 2010; 17(3):416–422

[28] Garcia MJ, Lookstein R, Malhotra R, et al. Endovascular management of deep vein thrombosis with rheolytic thrombectomy: final report of the prospective multicenter PEARL (Peripheral Use of AngioJet Rheolytic Thrombectomy with a Variety of Catheter Lengths) Registry. J Vasc Interv Radiol. 2015; 26(6):777–785, quiz 786

[29] Francis CW, Blinc A, Lee S, Cox C. Ultrasound accelerates transport of recombinant tissue plasminogen activator into clots. Ultrasound Med Biol. 1995; 21(3):419–424

[30] Garcia MJ. A treatment algorithm for DVT: determining therapeutic protocol for acute and chronic DVT. Endovascular Today. 2014; July:38–40

[31] Altman SD. A practical approach for diagnosis and treatment of central venous stenosis and occlusion. Semin Vasc Surg. 2007; 20(3):189–194

[32] Iafrati M, Maloney S, Halin N. Radiofrequency thermal wire is a useful adjunct to treat chronic central venous occlusions. J Vasc Surg. 2012; 55(2):603–606

[33] Guimaraes M, Schonholz C, Hannegan C, Anderson MB, Shi J, Selby B, Jr. Radiofrequency wire for the recanalization of central vein occlusions that have failed conventional endovascular techniques. J Vasc Interv Radiol. 2012; 23(8):1016–1021

[34] Kundu S, Modabber M, You JM, Tam P. Recanalization of chronic refractory central venous occlusions utilizing a radiofrequency guidewire perforation technique. J Vasc Access. 2012; 13(4):464–467

[35] Sivananthan G, MacArthur DH, Daly KP, Allen DW, Hakham S, Halin NJ. Safety and efficacy of radiofrequency wire recanalization of chronic central venous occlusions. J Vasc Access. 2015; 16(4):309–314

[36] Ferral H, Bjarnason H, Wholey M, Lopera J, Maynar M, Castaneda-Zuniga WR. Recanalization of occluded veins to provide access for central catheter placement. J Vasc Interv Radiol. 1996; 7(5):681–685

[37] Arabi M, Ahmed I, Mat'hami A, Ahmed D, Aslam N. Sharp central venous recanalization in hemodialysis patients: a single-institution experience. Cardiovasc Intervent Radiol. 2016; 39(6):927–934

[38] Nayak L, Hildebolt CF, Vedantham S. Postthrombotic syndrome: feasibility of a strategy of imaging-guided endovascular intervention. J Vasc Interv Radiol. 2012; 23(9):1165–1173

[39] Neglén P. Stenting is the "method-of-choice" to treat iliofemoral venous outflow obstruction. J Endovasc Ther. 2009; 16(4):492–493

[40] Raju S, Neglén P. Percutaneous recanalization of total occlusions of the iliac vein. J Vasc Surg. 2009; 50(2):360–368

[41] Hartung O, Otero A, Boufi M, et al. Mid-term results of endovascular treatment for symptomatic chronic nonmalignant iliocaval venous occlusive disease. J Vasc Surg. 2005; 42(6):1138–1144, discussion 1144

[42] Titus JM, Moise MA, Bena J, Lyden SP, Clair DG. Iliofemoral stenting for venous occlusive disease. J Vasc Surg. 2011; 53(3):706–712

[43] Raju S, Owen S, Jr, Neglen P. The clinical impact of iliac venous stents in the management of chronic venous insufficiency. J Vasc Surg. 2002; 35(1):8–15

[44] Neglén P, Raju S. Intravascular ultrasound scan evaluation of the obstructed vein. J Vasc Surg. 2002; 35(4):694–700

[45] Neglén P, Raju S. Balloon dilation and stenting of chronic iliac vein obstruction: technical aspects and early clinical outcome. J Endovasc Ther. 2000; 7(2):79–91

[46] Neglén P, Tackett TP, Jr, Raju S. Venous stenting across the inguinal ligament. J Vasc Surg. 2008; 48(5):1255–1261

[47] Ye K, Lu X, Jiang M, et al. Technical details and clinical outcomes of transpopliteal venous stent placement for postthrombotic chronic total occlusion of the iliofemoral vein. J Vasc Interv Radiol. 2014; 25(6):925–932

[48] Sista AK. Postprocedural management of patients undergoing endovascular therapy for acute and chronic lower-extremity deep venous disease. Tech Vasc Interv Radiol. 2014; 17(2):127–131

[49] Endo M, Jahangiri Y, Horikawa M, et al. Antiplatelet therapy is associated with stent patency after iliocaval venous stenting. Cardiovasc Intervent Radiol. 2018; 41(11):1691–1698

[50] Launois R, Reboul-Marty J, Henry B. Construction and validation of a quality of life questionnaire in chronic lower limb venous insufficiency (CIVIQ). Qual Life Res. 1996; 5(6):539–554

[51] Raju S. Best management options for chronic iliac vein stenosis and occlusion. J Vasc Surg. 2013; 57(4):1163–1169

[52] Sildiroglu O, Ozer H, Turba UC. Management of the thrombosed filter-bearing inferior vena cava. Semin Intervent Radiol. 2012; 29(1):57–63

[53] Ahmad I, Yeddula K, Wicky S, Kalva SP. Clinical sequelae of thrombus in an inferior vena cava filter. Cardiovasc Intervent Radiol. 2010; 33(2):285–289

[54] Hage AN, Srinivasa RN, Abramowitz SD, et al. Endovascular iliocaval reconstruction for the treatment of iliocaval thrombosis: from imaging to intervention. Vasc Med. 2018; 23(3):267–275

[55] Chick JFB, Jo A, Meadows JM, et al. Endovascular iliocaval stent reconstruction for inferior vena cava filter-associated iliocaval thrombosis: approach, technical success, safety, and two-year outcomes in 120 patients. J Vasc Interv Radiol. 2017; 28(7):933–939

[56] Chick JFB, Srinivasa RN, Cooper KJ, et al. Endovascular iliocaval reconstruction for chronic iliocaval thrombosis: the data, where we are, and how it is done. Tech Vasc Interv Radiol. 2018; 21(2):92–104

[57] Chiu KM, Chu SH, Chan CY. Dislodged caval stent in right pulmonary artery. Catheter Cardiovasc Interv. 2007; 70(6):799–800

[58] Dubois P, Mandieau A, Dolatabadi D, et al. Right ventricular migration of a stent after endovascular treatment of a superior vena cava syndrome. Arch Mal Coeur Vaiss. 2001; 94(11):1180–1183

[59] Egglin TK, Dickey KW, Rosenblatt M, Pollak JS. Retrieval of intravascular foreign bodies: experience in 32 cases. AJR Am J Roentgenol. 1995; 164(5):1259–1264

[60] Marcy PY, Magné N, Bruneton JN. Strecker stent migration to the pulmonary artery: long-term result of a "wait-and-see attitude." Eur Radiol. 2001; 11(5):767–770

[61] Gabelmann A, Krämer SC, Tomczak R, Görich J. Percutaneous techniques for managing maldeployed or migrated stents. J Endovasc Ther. 2001; 8(3):291–302

[62] Kölbel T, Lindh M, Akesson M, Wassèlius J, Gottsäter A, Ivancev K. Chronic iliac vein occlusion: midterm results of endovascular recanalization. J Endovasc Ther. 2009; 16(4):483–491

[63] Rosales A, Sandbaek G, Jørgensen JJ. Stenting for chronic post-thrombotic vena cava and iliofemoral venous occlusions: mid-term patency and clinical outcome. Eur J Vasc Endovasc Surg. 2010; 40(2):234–240

[64] Murphy EH, Johns B, Varney E, Raju S. Endovascular management of chronic total occlusions of the inferior vena cava and iliac veins. J Vasc Surg Venous Lymphat Disord. 2017; 5(1):47–59

[65] Neglén P, Hollis KC, Olivier J, Raju S. Stenting of the venous outflow in chronic venous disease: long-term stent-related outcome, clinical, and hemodynamic result. J Vasc Surg. 2007; 46(5):979–990

Chapter 9

Pulmonary Embolism

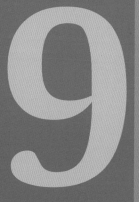

9 Pulmonary Embolism

Mina S. Makary, Alexander Y. Kim, Mamdouh Khayat, and Joshua D. Dowell

Keywords: pulmonary embolism, mechanical thrombectomy, lysis

9.1 Clinical Assessment: Massive versus Submassive

Most patients presenting with pulmonary embolism (PE) often have nonspecific symptoms such as dyspnea and chest pain, while some may experience pleuritic chest pain, tachycardia, fevers, and hemoptysis. Regardless of the presentation, the clinical evaluation of a patient presenting with acute PE should be centered on imaging findings and hemodynamic stability. Perfusion/ventilation nuclear medicine scans have been the diagnostic tool of choice to diagnose PE. This has largely been replaced in recent years with pulmonary computed tomography (CT) angiography due to its diagnostic accuracy, speed, clot burden assessment, and associated cardiac effects (▶ Fig. 9.1). The role of a diagnostic pulmonary angiography is limited due to its invasive nature but does allow for diagnostic confirmation and direct measurement of pulmonary arterial pressures prior to catheter-based treatment (▶ Fig. 9.2).

Once the diagnosis of PE is made, hemodynamic stability dictates treatment approaches and is generally used to stratify the PE as massive, submassive, or low risk.[1] Massive PE is defined by hemodynamic instability with systolic blood pressure < 90 mm Hg

for > 15 minutes or requiring inotropic support, cardiac arrest, pulselessness, or persistent profound bradycardia (< 40 beats per minute). In contrast, submassive PE is characterized by hemodynamic stability with a systolic blood pressure ≥ 90 mm Hg, but clinical evidence of right ventricular (RV) dysfunction including the right ventricle-to-left ventricle (RV/LV) ratio of > 0.9 on CT or echocardiogram (▶ Fig. 9.3), electrocardiogram changes, and/or laboratory values indicative of heart failure or myocardial injury. Stable, low-risk PE occurs in patients who are normotensive and are without RV dysfunction. The more severe the patient's presentation, including acute-onset hypotension, syncope, hypoxemia, or even cardiac arrest, the higher likelihood the PE is massive; therefore, higher clinical suspicion and prompt evaluation should be pursued.[1,2]

9.2 Medical/Systemic Treatment of PE: Anticoagulation and Thrombolysis

Anticoagulation is the core therapy for patients with acute PE. Anticoagulation agents are thought to "stabilize" thrombus and inhibit further propagation of the clot. It should be initiated immediately following the diagnosis of PE or empirically in the setting of high clinical suspicion for PE, unless a known contraindication is present. Systemic intravenous fractionated heparin, subcutaneous unfractionated low-molecular-weight heparin, or

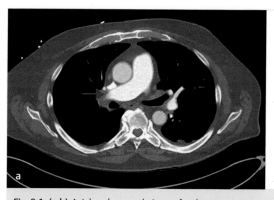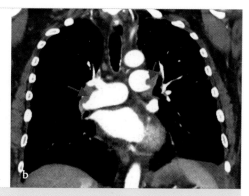

Fig. 9.1 (a,b) Axial and coronal views of pulmonary computed tomography angiography (CTA) demonstrating large central pulmonary emboli.

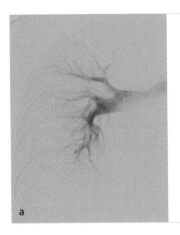 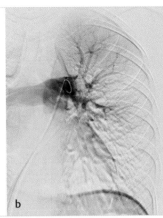

Fig. 9.2 (a,b) Pulmonary angiogram demonstrating central filling defects in bilateral pulmonary arteries consistent with pulmonary embolism.

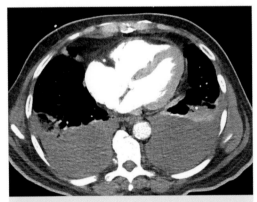

Fig. 9.3 Right ventricle-to-left ventricle (RV/LV) ratio > 0.9 in patient with bilateral pulmonary embolism (PE).

subcutaneous fondaparinux are the mainstay systemic therapies. Any of these agents is used to "bridge" patients while a concurrent oral anticoagulant agent such as warfarin reaches therapeutic levels.[3,4] Newer oral agents are also now available in the market and are often used as alternatives to warfarin including apixaban (Eliquis, Bristol-Myers Squibb/Pfizer), rivaroxaban (Xarelto, Janssen), edoxaban (Savaysa, Daiichi Sankyo), and dabigatran etexilate (Pradaxa, Boehringer Ingelheim).[5] Anticoagulant drug choice should be based on bleeding risk, reversal agent availability, and cost.[6] Anticoagulation alone is typically sufficient for patients with stable, low-risk PE.

For patients presenting with massive PE, thrombolytic agents have been shown to be more effective in diminishing clot burden compared to systemic

anticoagulants alone.[7] Unlike anticoagulants, which are used to prevent further thrombus formation, thrombolytics actively dissolve blood clots. These drugs cleave the inactive plasminogen into its active form: plasmin. Plasmin then breaks cross-links between fibrin molecules, which provide the underlying structure of blood clots. The most commonly used thrombolytic is tissue plasminogen activator (tPA), but other available U.S. Food and Drug Administration (FDA) approved thrombolytics for PE treatment include streptokinase, urokinase, and alteplase (Activase, Genentech).[5] Typically, the drug is administered as a peripheral intravenous infusion over a 2-hour period.[3,8] Per the latest guidelines by the American Heart Association (AHA), the American College of Chest Physicians (ACCP), the European Heart Association (EHA), and the American College of Emergency Physicians (ACEP), thrombolytic therapy is recommended for patients presenting with acute massive PE, which accounts for 5% of patients.[1,2,9,10,11]

The role of thrombolytics in submassive PE treatment remains a controversial point of debate. The multicenter, double-blind, placebo-controlled Pulmonary Embolism Thrombolysis Trial (PEITHO) trial assessed 1,005 patients with submassive PE treated with tenecteplase versus placebo along with unfractionated heparin. The study met its primary endpoint of demonstrating statistically significant decrease in all-cause mortality or hemodynamic decompensation (2.6 vs. 5.6%, $p = 0.02$), in favor of the tenecteplase group. However, tenecteplase use was associated with increased rates of major bleeding complication including intracranial hemorrhage (2.4 vs. 0.2%, $p = 0.004$). Other trials including Management Strategies and Prognosis of Pulmonary Embolism 3 (MAPPET3), Tenecteplase Italian Pulmonary Embolism Study (TIPES), and Tenecteplase or Placebo Cardiopulmonary Outcome at Three Months (TOPCOAT) demonstrated similarly equivocal data.[12,13,14,15,16] Given this, there is no clear consensus among society guidelines for the routine use of thrombolytic therapy in patients with submassive PE.[1,9,10,11] Treatment for this group of patients, which constitute a majority of those presenting with PE (31–64%), therefore should be determined on an individual basis in a multidisciplinary approach with consideration of the risks, benefits, and expected outcomes for the patient.[5,17]

9.3 Pharmacologic Catheter-Directed Lysis

9.3.1 Traditional vs. Ultrasound Assisted (EKOS)

Catheter-directed thrombolysis may have the advantage of reducing major bleeding complications compared with systemic administration. Traditional catheter-directed thrombolysis delivers the thrombolytic agent within thrombus via a catheter used to select a particular pulmonary artery (PA) or branch containing clot (▶ Fig. 9.4a). The rationale behind catheter-directed therapy is to increase the surface area of the thrombus exposed to the thrombolytic agent, which may allow for a lower dose of thrombolytics to be used.[7] Although this approach has not been shown to have better outcomes compared to systemic intravenous thrombolytic therapy,[7,18] there appears to be a lower level of serious bleeding events compared with systemic thrombolytic infusion. Catheter-directed thrombolysis may be particularly useful in patients who are higher bleeding risk, and the ACCP recommends its use in selected unstable patients who are unable to receive full-dose systemic thrombolysis.[10]

Standard catheter-directed regimens include continuous thrombolytic infusion for 12 to 48 hours. The thrombolytic agent is infused through a multiple–side hole catheter system. Several options are currently available including Uni-Fuse Pulse-Spray infusion catheter (AngioDynamics, Queensbury, NY), SpeedLyser Infusion System (AngioDynamics), Cragg-McNamara valved infusion catheter (Medtronic, Plymouth, MN), MicroMewi multiple side hole infusion catheter/microcatheter (Covidien, Dublin, Ireland), ProStream infusion wire (Covidien), Fountain infusion system (Merit Medical, South Jordan, UT), and Mistique infusion catheter (Merit Medical). tPA is administered unilaterally at a dose rate of 1.0 to 2.0 mg/hour or bilaterally with 0.5 to 1.0 mg/hour through each catheter.[19] Concurrent anticoagulation with heparin is recommended to prevent thrombus propagation. A typical initial heparin bolus is 2,000 to 5,000 units followed by a low-dose infusion of 100 to 500 units/hour.

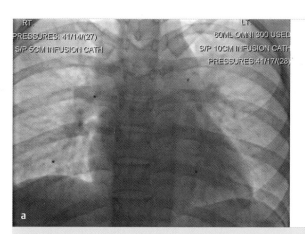
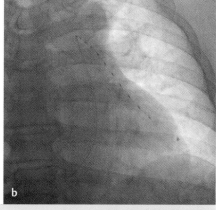

Fig. 9.4 (a) Fluoroscopic image of infusion catheters placed in bilateral pulmonary artery. Multiple side holes are located with a segment of catheter between the black marks. **(b)** Fluoroscopic image of an EkoSonic catheter in the left pulmonary artery.

Ultrasound-assisted thrombolysis is a novel development of conventional catheter-directed thrombolysis (▶ Fig. 9.4b). The EkoSonic Endovascular System is the only endovascular device approved by the FDA in this category. This treatment approach utilizes high-frequency low-energy ultrasound waves that do not directly break down the thrombus, but rather augment the thrombolytic drug by increasing clot permeability through disaggregation of uncrosslinked fibrin fibers.[20,21] The safety and efficacy of EkoSonic catheter was studied in the Submassive and Massive Pulmonary Embolism Treatment with Ultrasound Accelerated Thrombolysis Therapy (SEATTLE-2) trial, a prospective, multicenter, single-arm study of 150 patients with acute massive or submassive PE. A statistically significant improvement was demonstrated in the mean RV/LV ratio (1.55 vs. 1.13; $p < 0.0001$) and mean PA systolic pressures (51.4 vs. 36.9 mm Hg; $p < 0.0001$) versus baseline. Moderate bleeding events were seen in 15 patients (10%) and there were no incidents of intracranial hemorrhage. In comparison with the traditional pharmacologic catheter-directed thrombolysis, this ultrasound-assisted approach offers similar treatment outcomes with possibly reduced infusion time and bleeding complications.[22] This therapy further reduces thrombolytic drug dosage requirements compared to the traditional catheter-directed approach.[23]

9.3.2 Contraindications/Cautions

Several contraindications for catheter-directed thrombolysis should be considered and cautiously evaluated prior to interventions. Major contraindications include evidence of active bleeding, bleeding disorder, history of intracranial bleeding, ischemic stroke within 3 months, recent brain or spine surgery, and metastatic disease to the brain. Relative contraindications include an age greater than 75 years, low body weight (<60 kg), traumatic cardiopulmonary resuscitation (CPR; e.g., prolonged chest compressions), systolic blood pressure > 180 mm Hg, diastolic blood pressure > 110 mm Hg, current anticoagulation, pregnancy, pericarditis, recent surgery or invasive procedure within 10 days, and recent major nonintracranial bleeding.[4,10] An additional consideration is an allergic reaction to the thrombolytic agent, particularly streptokinase, which has been described in up to 16% of patients.[24] These contraindications should likewise be considered in the setting of anticoagulation and systemic thrombolysis.

9.3.3 Patient Monitoring

Close patient monitoring is paramount following initiation of thrombolysis therapy. Patients should be placed on strict bedrest. Monitoring for occult hemorrhage, including serial neurologic examinations should be performed routinely. Palpating distal limb pulses for early signs of distal embolism is recommended. Routine assessment of coagulation status is obtained every 4 to 6 hours—a peripherally inserted central catheter (PICC) may be placed prior to initiation of thrombolysis to prevent repeated peripheral venous punctures. Partial thromboplastin time (PTT) should be maintained at 1.5 to 2.5 times the normal limits, indicating therapeutic heparinization. Assessment of fibrinogen levels is controversial; however, many interventional radiologists choose to monitor patients during thrombolysis to reduce the risk of major hemorrhage. Target levels are often institution based, but one standard practice is to reduce the infusion rate when fibrinogen levels drop below 50% of prior value and held if less than 100 mg/dL.[19]

9.3.4 Mechanical Thrombectomy

To help debulk and expedite clearance of thrombus burden from acutely occluded segments, physical fragmentation by percutaneous mechanical thrombectomy devices can be considered.[25,26] Mechanical thrombolysis is often considered for patients with large central thrombus burden. The combination of thrombus aspiration, maceration, and dissolution functions to more promptly fragment clots to reduce life-threatening heart strain and improve pulmonary perfusion. Fragmentation also exposes more thrombus surface area to the effects of locally infused thrombolytic drugs; thus, mechanical thrombolysis is often followed by thrombolytic infusion.[27] The technology of mechanical thrombectomy devices continues to expand and can be categorically divided into three subgroups: aspiration, rotational, and hydrodynamic.

9.3.5 Aspiration Thrombectomy

Manual aspiration can be performed through any end-hole catheter through an appropriately sized sheath. This method is ideal for more central clot burden, and can often be used in conjunction with other debulking techniques. A syringe is employed to suction and aspirate clot through the catheter.[28]

AngioVac (AngioDynamics, Latham, NY) is a motorized device that functions to eradicate thrombus by aspirating using an extracorporeal filtering system that eliminates clot debris and recirculates blood to the patient. Few reports are published on the utilization of AngioVac in pulmonary emboli and more research needs to be conducted on its potential role in the treatment of this patient population.

A newer device, the Inari FlowTriever (Inari Medical, Irvine, CA) allows for manual aspiration of clot through a flexible, large-bore catheter using a proprietary large-bore syringe. Fragmentation of the clot occurs through rapid application of suction and/or the use of three self-expanding nitinol disks that can be introduced through the catheter and used to pull clot into the aspiration catheter.

9.3.6 Rotational Devices

Rotational thrombectomy devices utilize a high-speed rotating impeller or basket lattice to macerate the thrombus. There is a theoretical risk that the macerated particles can travel distally into the pulmonary circulation with resultant elevation in pulmonary arterial pressures, requiring adjuvant therapies to complete treatment.[29] A common technique is utilization of a rotating pigtail to fragment the thrombus. The catheter can be rotated manually or electronically with a motor attached to the catheter hub. The side holes of the distal pigtail can be employed to infuse thrombolytic drugs directly into the thrombus.[30]

Alternatively, a high rotation per minute (RPM) rotational device like the Helix Clot Buster (ev3/ Covidien, Plymouth, MN), formerly known as the *Amplatz thrombectomy device* (ATD), can be used to debulk pulmonary emboli. This device is a 7-Fr catheter with a distal metal tip containing an impeller that can generate up to 140,000 RPM during operation with concurrent active aspiration. These devices do not run over a wire and care must be taken to avoid vascular injury.[31,32]

9.3.7 Hydrodynamic Devices

In hydrodynamic or rheolytic thrombectomy, a high-pressure saline jet functions to fragment thrombus in conjunction with aspiration and thus create the Venturi effect. An example of a hydrodynamic recirculation device is the Hydrolyzer (Cordis) catheter, a 6- to 7-Fr double-lumen catheter with a distal atraumatic tip and a more proximal side hole. A single, high-speed retrograde fluid jet is directed through the side hole, generating the Venturi effect and fragmenting the thrombus and directing it into the distal evacuation lumen. One study demonstrated a 70 to 75% reduction of centrally located thrombus with a decrease in pulmonary arterial hypertension and RV strain.[33]

The AngioJet Xpeedior thrombectomy device is a 4- to 6-Fr over-the-wire catheter that utilizes the Venturi effect to induce thrombus aspiration. Moreover, it permits concomitant infusion of thrombolytics to expedite thrombus dissolution. Although widely employed for deep venous thrombi, its utilization in pulmonary vasculature is controversial given a higher procedural complication rate.[34] Multiple deaths related to the AngioJet have been documented in the FDA's MAUDE (Manufacturer and User Facility Device Experience) database, prompting the FDA to issue a black box warning on the device.[35]

9.3.8 Surgical Thrombectomy

Historically, pulmonary endarterectomy has been pursued in unstable patients with massive pulmonary embolus or patients with contraindication to catheter-directed thrombolysis. Recent improvements in operative technique have decreased the perioperative mortality rate to 4.4%.[36] It can be performed in the treatment of chronic pulmonary hypertension from thrombotic disease.[37] A study by Riedel et al demonstrated that patients with PA pressure more than 30 mm Hg had a 30% 5-year survival. This deteriorated to 10% survival at 5 years if pressures were elevated beyond 50 mm Hg.[38,39] Pulmonary thromboendarterectomy may lead to improved long-term outcomes, with one study demonstrating a 6-year survival rate of 75% in selected patients.[36]

References

[1] Jaff MR, McMurtry MS, Archer SL, et al. American Heart Association Council on Cardiopulmonary, Critical Care, Perioperative and Resuscitation, American Heart Association Council on Peripheral Vascular Disease, American Heart Association Council on Arteriosclerosis, Thrombosis and Vascular Biology. Management of massive and submassive pulmonary embolism, iliofemoral deep vein thrombosis, and chronic thromboembolic pulmonary hypertension: a scientific statement from the American Heart Association. Circulation. 2011; 123 (16):1788–1830

[2] Pelliccia F, Schiariti M, Terzano C, et al. Treatment of acute pulmonary embolism: update on newer pharmacologic and interventional strategies. BioMed Res Int. 2014; 2014: 410341

[3] Banovac F, Buckley DC, Kuo WT, et al. Technology Assessment Committee of the Society of Interventional Radiology. Reporting standards for endovascular treatment of pulmonary embolism. J Vasc Interv Radiol. 2010; 21(1):44–53

[4] Saad N. Aggressive management of pulmonary embolism. Semin Intervent Radiol. 2012; 29(1):52–56

[5] Martin C, Sobolewski K, Bridgeman P, Boutsikaris D. Systemic thrombolysis for pulmonary embolism: a review. P&T. 2016; 41(12):770–775

[6] Streiff MB, Agnelli G, Connors JM, et al. Guidance for the treatment of deep vein thrombosis and pulmonary embolism. J Thromb Thrombolysis. 2016; 41(1):32–67

[7] De Gregorio MA, Gimeno MJ, Mainar A, et al. Mechanical and enzymatic thrombolysis for massive pulmonary embolism. J Vasc Interv Radiol. 2002; 13(2, Pt 1):163–169

[8] Carson JL, Kelley MA, Duff A, et al. The clinical course of pulmonary embolism. N Engl J Med. 1992; 326(19):1240–1245

[9] Torbicki A, Perrier A, Konstantinides S, et al. ESC Committee for Practice Guidelines (CPG). Guidelines on the diagnosis and management of acute pulmonary embolism: the Task Force for the Diagnosis and Management of Acute Pulmonary Embolism of the European Society of Cardiology (ESC). Eur Heart J. 2008; 29(18):2276–2315

[10] Kearon C, Akl EA, Ornelas J, et al. Antithrombotic therapy for VTE disease: CHEST Guideline and Expert Panel Report. Chest. 2016; 149(2):315–352

[11] Fesmire FM, Brown MD, Espinosa JA, et al. American College of Emergency Physicians. Critical issues in the evaluation and management of adult patients presenting to the emergency department with suspected pulmonary embolism. Ann Emerg Med. 2011; 57(6):628–652.e75

[12] Konstantinides S, Geibel A, Heusel G, Heinrich F, Kasper W, Management Strategies and Prognosis of Pulmonary Embolism-3 Trial Investigators. Heparin plus alteplase compared with heparin alone in patients with submassive pulmonary embolism. N Engl J Med. 2002; 347(15):1143–1150

[13] Sharifi M, Bay C, Skrocki L, Rahimi F, Mehdipour M, "MOPETT" Investigators. Moderate pulmonary embolism treated with thrombolysis (from the "MOPETT" trial). Am J Cardiol. 2013; 111(2):273–277

[14] Meyer G, Vicaut E, Danays T, et al. PEITHO Investigators. Fibrinolysis for patients with intermediate-risk pulmonary embolism. N Engl J Med. 2014; 370(15):1402–1411

[15] Becattini C, Agnelli G, Salvi A, et al. TIPES Study Group. Bolus tenecteplase for right ventricle dysfunction in hemodynamically stable patients with pulmonary embolism. Thromb Res. 2010; 125(3):e82–e86

[16] Kline JA, Nordenholz KE, Courtney DM, et al. Treatment of submassive pulmonary embolism with tenecteplase or placebo: cardiopulmonary outcomes at 3 months: multicenter double-blind, placebo-controlled randomized trial. J Thromb Haemost. 2014; 12(4):459–468

[17] Grifoni S, Olivotto I, Cecchini P, et al. Short-term clinical outcome of patients with acute pulmonary embolism, normal blood pressure, and echocardiographic right ventricular dysfunction. Circulation. 2000; 101(24):2817–2822

[18] Verstraete M, Miller GA, Bounameaux H, et al. Intravenous and intrapulmonary recombinant tissue-type plasminogen activator in the treatment of acute massive pulmonary embolism. Circulation. 1988; 77(2):353–360

[19] Kuo WT. Endovascular therapy for acute pulmonary embolism. J Vasc Interv Radiol. 2012; 23(2):167–179.e4, quiz 179

[20] Gaba RC, Gundavaram MS, Parvinian A, et al. Efficacy and safety of flow-directed pulmonary artery catheter thrombolysis for treatment of submassive pulmonary embolism. AJR Am J Roentgenol. 2014; 202(6):1355–1360

[21] Braaten JV, Goss RA, Francis CW. Ultrasound reversibly disaggregates fibrin fibers. Thromb Haemost. 1997; 78(3):1063–1068

[22] Mostafa A, Briasoulis A, Telila T, Belgrave K, Grines C. Treatment of massive or submassive acute pulmonary embolism with catheter-directed thrombolysis. Am J Cardiol. 2016; 117(6):1014–1020

[23] Parikh S, Motarjeme A, McNamara T, et al. Ultrasound-accelerated thrombolysis for the treatment of deep vein thrombosis: initial clinical experience. J Vasc Interv Radiol. 2008; 19(4):521–528

[24] Zeni PT, Jr, Blank BG, Peeler DW. Use of rheolytic thrombectomy in treatment of acute massive pulmonary embolism. J Vasc Interv Radiol. 2003; 14(12):1511–1515

[25] Frisoli JK, Sze D. Mechanical thrombectomy for the treatment of lower extremity deep vein thrombosis. Tech Vasc Interv Radiol. 2003; 6(1):49–52

[26] Sharafuddin MJ, Sun S, Hoballah JJ, Youness FM, Sharp WJ, Roh BS. Endovascular management of venous thrombotic and occlusive diseases of the lower extremities. J Vasc Interv Radiol. 2003; 14(4):405–423

[27] Kuo WT, Gould MK, Louie JD, Rosenberg JK, Sze DY, Hofmann LV. Catheter-directed therapy for the treatment of massive pulmonary embolism: systematic review and meta-analysis of modern techniques. J Vasc Interv Radiol. 2009; 20(11):1431–1440

[28] Lang EV, Barnhart WH, Walton DL, Raab SS. Percutaneous pulmonary thrombectomy. J Vasc Interv Radiol. 1997; 8(3):427–432

[29] Nakazawa K, Tajima H, Murata S, Kumita SI, Yamamoto T, Tanaka K. Catheter fragmentation of acute massive pulmonary thromboembolism: distal embolisation and pulmonary arterial pressure elevation. Br J Radiol. 2008; 81(971):848–854

[30] Schmitz-Rode T, Janssens U, Duda SH, Erley CM, Günther RW. Massive pulmonary embolism: percutaneous emergency treatment by pigtail rotation catheter. J Am Coll Cardiol. 2000; 36(2):375–380

[31] Uflacker R, Strange C, Vujic I. Massive pulmonary embolism: preliminary results of treatment with the Amplatz thrombectomy device. J Vasc Interv Radiol. 1996; 7(4):519–528

[32] Rocek M, Peregrin J, Velimsky T. Mechanical thrombectomy of massive pulmonary embolism using an Arrow-Trerotola percutaneous thrombolytic device. Eur Radiol. 1998; 8(9):1683–1685

[33] Fava M, Loyola S, Huete I. Massive pulmonary embolism: treatment with the hydrolyser thrombectomy catheter. J Vasc Interv Radiol. 2000; 11(9):1159–1164

[34] Kuo WT, Sze DY, Hofmann LV. Catheter-directed intervention for acute pulmonary embolism: a shining saber. Chest. 2008; 133(1):317–318, author reply 318

[35] AngioJet Xpeedior [product insert]. Minneapolis, MN: Possis Medical; 2008

[36] Jamieson SW, Kapelanski DP, Sakakibara N, et al. Pulmonary endarterectomy: experience and lessons learned in 1,500 cases. Ann Thorac Surg. 2003; 76(5):1457–1462, discussion 1462–1464

[37] Mo M, Kapelanski DP, Mitruka SN, et al. Reoperative pulmonary thromboendarterectomy. Ann Thorac Surg. 1999; 68(5):1770–1776, discussion 1776–1777

[38] Jamieson SW, Kapelanski DP. Pulmonary endarterectomy. Curr Probl Surg. 2000; 37(3):165–252

[39] Riedel M, Stanek V, Widimsky J, Prerovsky I. Longterm follow-up of patients with pulmonary thromboembolism. Late prognosis and evolution of hemodynamic and respiratory data. Chest. 1982; 81(2):151–158

Chapter 10

Venous Thromboembolism: Management of Bleeding Complications

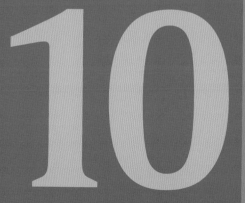

10 Venous Thromboembolism: Management of Bleeding Complications

James Chen and Deepak Sudheendra

10.1 Bleeding Complications Associated with Venous Thromboembolism Treatment

The treatment of venous thromboembolism (VTE) remains challenging and limitations to conventional treatment with systemic anticoagulation (AC) have led to the advent of catheter-directed thrombolysis (CDT) and pharmacomechanical CDT (PCDT) techniques, which more rapidly decrease clot burden and decrease the severity and rate of long-term sequelae such as postthrombotic syndrome (PTS) following deep vein thrombosis (DVT).[1,2] Both CDT and PCDT involve placement of an infusion catheter into a clot for local infusion of thrombolytic, with adjunctive techniques for thrombus removal including rheolytic systems for thromboaspiration in PCDT. Local thrombolytic infusion allows for higher local doses with less systemic exposure, affording decreased bleeding complications compared to systemic thrombolytic administration. A variety of fibrinolytics are available, such as tissue plasminogen activator (tPA) and streptokinase, all of which function by activation of plasmin, which facilitates clot lysis by fibrin degradation. Although refinements of CDT and PCDT techniques and thrombolytic agents over the past few decades have afforded improved complication profiles, there remains an elevated risk of major bleeding when using these therapies compared to systemic AC alone.

The pathophysiologies of bleeding complications during CDT/PCDT are related to a combination of thrombolytic mechanisms including plasmin-mediated degradation of fibrin, reduced plasma concentrations of fibrinogen and other clotting factors, and antiplatelet effects. Although the half-lives of thrombolytic drugs are short (i.e., tPA has a half-life of 5 minutes), the associated depletion of clotting cascade factors and antiplatelet effects leads to prolonged coagulopathic effects after cessation of infusion. Fibrinogen levels, for instance, require up to 48 hours to return to baseline levels after stopping thrombolytics. When bleeding complications occur, a large majority of the complications are venous access site–related minor bleeding episodes, which can typically be managed conservatively and do not result in long-term sequelae. Major bleeding, defined as bleeding resulting in hemodynamic compromise or intracranial hemorrhage (ICH), occurs in a small minority of cases, ranging from 2 to 3% in most modern studies.[2,3,4,5,6,7] A Cochrane analysis of CDT studies found that all cases of ICH occurred in pre-1990 studies[8] and a meta-analysis of pulmonary embolism (PE) thrombolysis reported a 0.35% rate of ICH.[9]

10.1.1 Patient Selection and Monitoring for Bleeding Complications

Although the risk of major bleeding is low, the potentially catastrophic nature of these episodes necessitates judicious patient selection for CDT/PCDT. The following absolute contraindications to CDT/PCDT have been suggested by guidelines from the Society of Interventional Radiology (SIR)[7]:

- Active internal bleeding or disseminated intravascular coagulation (DIC).
- Recent cerebrovascular accident (CVA), neurosurgery, or intracranial trauma (within 3 months).
- Absolute contraindication to AC.

During placement of the infusion catheter, ultrasound-guided venous access with a micropuncture set should be used to decrease the number of puncture attempts and reduce the risk of access site bleeding complications.[7] No arterial or intramuscular injections should be administered and no additional venous access should be attempted during thrombolysis due to bleeding risk.

The recommended tPA infusion rate for VTE is 0.01 mg/kg/hour, not to exceed 1.0 mg/hour. Concurrent AC is typically attained using heparin drip or low-molecular-weight heparin (LMWH).[10] For patients receiving heparin drip, target partial thromboplastin time (PTT) is controversial, with some groups advocating a subtherapeutic PTT target of 1.2 to 1.7 times control,[2] based on studies demonstrating elevated bleeding risk with therapeutic PTT targets.[11] At our institution, we administer enoxaparin (Lovenox) 1 mg/kg at full AC dose. We have found that this protocol allows greater ease of achieving steady-state AC, and eliminates the frequent PTT checks required with heparin drip. Patients with heparin-induced thrombocytopenia (HIT) should undergo AC with a direct thrombin inhibitor such as argatroban or bivalirudin. Patients undergoing CDT require bedrest with immobilization of the catheter-bearing limb, and vigilant clinical evaluation for any signs of impending major bleeding including acute mental status change, severe headache or abdominal pain, epistaxis, or other sentinel bleeding event. Serial laboratory evaluation of hemoglobin, PTT, and platelet levels is performed every 6 hours at our institution. The value of monitoring fibrinogen levels remains controversial, with conflicting evidence on the association between low fibrinogen level (< 1–1.5 g/L) and higher bleeding risk. An early trial citing the higher risk of bleeding with low fibrinogen levels was confounded by the use of therapeutic rather than subtherapeutic heparin doses,[11] and other studies have demonstrated discordant results in both venous and arterial thrombolysis settings.[12,13,14,15] In the absence of definitive data, society guidelines still recommend fibrinogen level monitoring,[7] and some groups advocate slowing down thrombolytic infusion rate once fibrinogen level is < 1.5 g/L and stopping the infusion completely once fibrinogen level is < 1.0 g/L.[14] At our institution, we do not routinely monitor fibrinogen levels. Higher thrombolytic doses and longer duration of infusion are associated with significantly higher risks of bleeding complication.[14]

10.1.2 Management of Bleeding Complications

Once a major bleeding episode is identified, the fibrinolytic and heparin infusions should be stopped immediately, and hemodynamic resuscitation should be initiated. The half-life of tPA is approximately 5 minutes. Laboratory evaluation of hemoglobin, platelet, international normalized ratio (INR), PTT, and fibrinogen levels should be attained. Depending on the laboratory findings, the patient may require blood products including fresh frozen plasma (FFP), cryoprecipitate, fibrinogen concentrate, platelets, and packed red blood cell transfusion. Some groups also administer tranexamic acid, an antifibrinolytic agent, for cases of severe hemorrhage, although in most cases, the 5-minute half-life of tPA is short enough that cessation of the infusion should be

sufficient. Protamine can be administered for rapid reversal of heparin AC at a dose of 10 mg for every 100 U of heparin, with a maximum dose of 50 mg. Given the emergent nature of major bleeding complications in the setting CDT/PCDT, there is a paucity of evidence on optimal management algorithm, and specific protocols vary between providers and institutions.[16,17] Persistent bleeding may require more aggressive interventions including embolization. The management of ICH is outside of the scope of this chapter, but includes optimization of intracranial pressure, blood pressure, and respiratory status. It is important to differentiate hematuria from periprocedural hemoglobinuria, which occurs commonly following PCDT with rheolytic thrombectomy, and will typically resolve in 24 to 32 hours. Minor bleeding episodes such as pericatheter oozing can be managed conservatively with manual compression.

10.1.3 Summary

Although the rate of major bleeding during CDT/PCDT for VTE is low, careful patient selection and vigilant monitoring during thrombolysis are essential to identify and mitigate the morbidity from these bleeding episodes. Once major bleeding is identified, thrombolytic and AC infusions should be immediately stopped, and resuscitation with coagulation factors and blood products may be required. Serial monitoring of fibrinogen levels remains an area of controversy, with conflicting evidence regarding the need to reduce or cease thrombolytic infusion at lower fibrinogen levels.

References

[1] Sharifi M, Bay C, Mehdipour M, Sharifi J, TORPEDO Investigators. Thrombus Obliteration by Rapid Percutaneous Endovenous Intervention in Deep Venous Occlusion (TORPEDO) trial: midterm results. J Endovasc Ther. 2012; 19(2):273–280

[2] Enden T, Haig Y, Kløw NE, et al. CaVenT Study Group. Long-term outcome after additional catheter-directed thrombolysis versus standard treatment for acute iliofemoral deep vein thrombosis (the CaVenT study): a randomised controlled trial. Lancet. 2012; 379(9810):31–38

[3] Enden T, Kløw NE, Sandvik L, et al. CaVenT study group. Catheter-directed thrombolysis vs. anticoagulant therapy alone in deep vein thrombosis: results of an open randomized, controlled trial reporting on short-term patency. J Thromb Haemost. 2009; 7(8):1268–1275

[4] Enden T, Wik HS, Kvam AK, Haig Y, Kløw NE, Sandset PM. Health-related quality of life after catheter-directed thrombolysis for deep vein thrombosis: secondary outcomes of the randomised, non-blinded, parallel-group CaVenT study. BMJ Open. 2013; 3(8):e002984

[5] Elsharawy M, Elzayat E. Early results of thrombolysis vs anti-coagulation in iliofemoral venous thrombosis. A randomised clinical trial. Eur J Vasc Endovasc Surg. 2002; 24(3):209–214

[6] Engelberger RP, Spirk D, Willenberg T, et al. Ultrasound-assisted versus conventional catheter-directed thrombolysis for acute iliofemoral deep vein thrombosis. Circ Cardiovasc Interv. 2015; 8(1):e002027

[7] Vedantham S, Sista AK, Klein SJ, et al. Society of Interventional Radiology and Cardiovascular and Interventional Radiological Society of Europe Standards of Practice Committees. Quality improvement guidelines for the treatment of lower-extremity deep vein thrombosis with use of endovascular thrombus removal. J Vasc Interv Radiol. 2014; 25(9):1317–1325

[8] Watson L, Broderick C, Armon MP. Thrombolysis for acute deep vein thrombosis. Cochrane Database Syst Rev. 2016; 11 (11):CD002783

[9] Bloomer TL, El-Hayek GE, McDaniel MC, et al. Safety of catheter-directed thrombolysis for massive and submassive pulmonary embolism: results of a multicenter registry and meta-analysis. Catheter Cardiovasc Interv. 2017; 89(4):754–760

[10] Foegh P, Jensen LP, Klitfod L, Broholm R, Bækgaard N. Editor's choice: factors associated with long-term outcome in 191 patients with ilio-femoral DVT treated with catheter-directed thrombolysis. Eur J Vasc Endovasc Surg. 2017; 53(3):419–424

[11] Ouriel K, Veith FJ, Sasahara AA, Thrombolysis or Peripheral Arterial Surgery (TOPAS) Investigators. A comparison of recombinant urokinase with vascular surgery as initial treatment for acute arterial occlusion of the legs. N Engl J Med. 1998; 338(16):1105–1111

[12] Results of a prospective randomized trial evaluating surgery versus thrombolysis for ischemia of the lower extremity. The STILE trial. Ann Surg. 1994; 220(3):251–266, discussion 266–268

[13] Skeik N, Gits CC, Ehrenwald E, Cragg AH. Fibrinogen level as a surrogate for the outcome of thrombolytic therapy using tissue plasminogen activator for acute lower extremity intra-vascular thrombosis. Vasc Endovascular Surg. 2013; 47(7): 519–523

[14] Lee K, Istl A, Dubois L, et al. Fibrinogen level and bleeding risk during catheter-directed thrombolysis using tissue plasminogen activator. Vasc Endovascular Surg. 2015; 49 (7):175–179

[15] Ouriel K, Kandarpa K, Schuerr DM, Hultquist M, Hodkinson G, Wallin B. Prourokinase versus urokinase for recanalization of peripheral occlusions, safety and efficacy: the PURPOSE trial. J Vasc Interv Radiol. 1999; 10(8):1083–1091

[16] Makris M, Van Veen JJ, Tait CR, Mumford AD, Laffan M, British Committee for Standards in Haematology. Guideline on the management of bleeding in patients on antithrombotic agents. Br J Haematol. 2013; 160(1):35–46

[17] Rasler F. Emergency treatment of hemorrhagic complications of thrombolysis. Ann Emerg Med. 2007; 50(4):485

10.2 Quality Improvement and Safety of Treatment of Thromboembolic Disease and Guidelines and Complication Thresholds for Treatment of DVT and PE

Boris Nikolic

The risks associated with deep vein thrombosis (DVT) are considerable and include pulmonary embolism (PE), postthrombotic syndrome, paradoxical (functionally patent foramen ovale–related) embolization, or limb or life loss due to venous gangrene and congestion with potentially massive fluid sequestration that may lead to circulatory collapse (phlegmasia cerulea dolens). Although clinical information is not always reliable, a dichotomization into acute and Chronic DVT based on DVT presence of less than or more than 3 weeks, respectively, is scientifically well grounded in histopathological findings. As with any treatment, therapeutic success is dependent upon diagnostic accuracy. Acute DVTs are not always distinguishable from chronic DVTs based on clinical history and acute on chronic manifestations may occur. As such, initiation of thrombolysis that is not primarily or that is incompletely successful may guide the interventional operator to acknowledge the presence of chronic thrombus and to proceed with mechanical recanalization and venous stent placement. Furthermore, it is important to recognize distinct underlying pathologies, such as May–Thurner (Cockett's) syndrome, venous compression by tumor, or hypercoagulable states, and to address those specifically as indicated and feasible.[1] This author generally advocates for the existence of institutional, evidence-based treatment algorithms, including one for patients referred for endovascular therapy of DVT and meeting such criteria, as exemplified in ► Fig. 10.1.

Endovascular venous thrombus removal can occur with pharmacological (systemic thrombolysis, flow-directed thrombolysis, catheter-directed intra-thrombus thrombolysis) or mechanical means (clot pulverization), but a combined pharmacomechanical approach is often the preferred one, where mechanical clot pulverization increases the exposed clot target surface area for plasminogen-activated thrombolysis, thus reducing hospital and ICU stay. In considering the indication for endovascular treatment of acute DVT, assessment of clinical severity is of particular relevance. The ATTRACT (Acute Venous Thrombosis: Thrombus Removal with Adjunctive Catheter-Directed Thrombolysis) trial (currently unpublished data)—largely considered sentinel in addressing the topic of approaching therapy of acute DVT—failed to show the superiority of endovascular treatment compared to systemic treatment in reducing future development of postthrombotic syndrome or in lowering treatment-related adverse event rates. Consequently, an interventional approach would generally not be justified in asymptomatic patients, which more commonly have thrombus limited to the femoropopliteal system. However, in severely symptomatic patients and in those with acutely threatened limbs—where iliac venous system

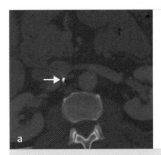 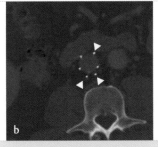 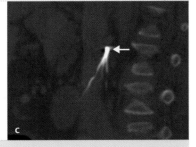

Fig. 10.1 Axial **(a)** and coronal **(b)** computed tomography images demonstrating peripheral calcifications of the lower IVC And iliac veins as sequalae of chronic venous occlusion. **(c)** coronal computed tomography images demonstrating the top of the filter penetrating outside of the caval wall (arrow).
Source: *Samuel M, Nahab B, Chadalavada S. Balloon-assisted retrieval of a retained vascular sheath during complex inferior vena cava filter removal. Semin Intervent Radiol. 2023; 40(3):298–303.*

involvement is typical—endovascular therapy is preferable over open surgical treatment.[2,3,4]

The most common major adverse event associated with endovascular treatment of DVT is substantial bleeding—with its intracranial manifestation being most feared.[5] Occurrence of symptomatic PE has also been reported. Frequency and severity of adverse events can often be reduced with proper patient selection and properly rigorous intra- and periprocedural monitoring. With regard to the former, patients with absolute contraindications, that is, active internal hemorrhage, recent stroke, transient ischemic attack (TIA) or cerebral trauma, or absolute contraindication to anticoagulation, should be excluded from thrombolysis considerations. With regard to the latter, initial micropuncture set venous access, a recombinant tissue plasminogen activator dose of < 1 mg/h, presence of frequent nurse-to-patient contact, monitoring of fibrinogen levels, immobilization of the punctured extremity, avoidance of stand-alone mechanical thrombolysis, and assurance of subtherapeutic effects of any anticoagulants that had previously been administered to the patient lower the risk profile for the occurrence of adverse events.[6,7]

Procedural efficacy outcome has been measured based on removal of > 50% of thrombus resulting in restoration of iliofemoral flow and absence of early (1–3 months postprocedural) thrombosis recurrence.[7] Corresponding practice thresholds for both parameters, below which an internal investigation should be considered, have been set by the Standards of Practice Committee of the Society of Interventional Radiology (SIR) as 80% each, provided that intrathrombus thrombolytic therapy occurred, treated thrombus was predominantly acute, heparin-based therapy could be administered during catheter manipulation and postprocedure completion, and that underlying flow-limiting stenoses were appropriately therapeutically addressed with venoplasty or stent placement.[8,9,10,11,12]

As for any complex interventional procedure, care is incomplete and inadequate without postprocedural clinical follow-up. In the case of endovascular DVT therapy, this entails at least two follow-up clinic visits with evaluation for postthrombotic syndrome (in > 80% of patients), postprocedural administration of anticoagulation for at least 3 months if DVT was related to a major initiating event (e.g., major surgery, trauma, etc.) and for 6 months in the absence of such event as well as arrangements for inferior vena cava (IVC) filter removal, if placed intraprocedurally. With regard to the latter, it is notable, however, that procedure-related PE is uncommon[9] and the appropriateness of IVC filter placement is therefore unclear.[13] Longer-term postprocedural (i.e., 2-year-long) application of elastic compression stockings has not proven more effective than placebo in more recent investigation but may be beneficial for more rapid reduction of swelling during the initial postprocedural weeks and for longer-term postthrombotic syndrome management in individual patients.[14]

In summary, a distinction between mostly acute and mostly chronic presence of DVT fundamentally impacts the type of treatment and endovascular technique. Patients with acute DVT, where endovascular management is considered, should be carefully selected, well monitored periprocedurally, and rigorously followed clinically for outcome. Based on most recent data, a highly symptomatic and threatened limb seems to present the most convincing indication for endovascular intervention.

References

[1] Goldman RE, Arendt VA, Kothary N, et al. Endovascular management of May-Thurner syndrome in adolescents: a single-center experience. J Vasc Interv Radiol. 2017; 28(1): 71–77
[2] Patel NH, Plorde JJ, Meissner M. Catheter-directed thrombolysis in the treatment of phlegmasia cerulea dolens. Ann Vasc Surg. 1998; 12(5):471–475
[3] Weaver FA, Meacham PW, Adkins RB, Dean RH. Phlegmasia cerulea dolens: therapeutic considerations. South Med J. 1988; 81(3):306–312
[4] Robinson DL, Teitelbaum GP. Phlegmasia cerulea dolens: treatment by pulse-spray and infusion thrombolysis. AJR Am J Roentgenol. 1993; 160(6):1288–1290
[5] Patel N, Sacks D, Patel RI, et al. Technology Assessment Committee of the Society of Cardiovascular & Interventioanal Radiology. SCVIR reporting standards for the treatment of acute limb ischemia with use of transluminal removal of arterial thrombus. J Vasc Interv Radiol. 2001; 12(5):559–570
[6] Uflacker R. Mechanical thrombectomy in acute and subacute thrombosis with use of the Amplatz device: arterial and venous applications. J Vasc Interv Radiol. 1997; 8(6):923–932
[7] Delomez M, Beregi JP, Willoteaux S, et al. Mechanical thrombectomy in patients with deep venous thrombosis. Cardiovasc Intervent Radiol. 2001; 24(1):42–48
[8] Mewissen MW, Seabrook GR, Meissner MH, Cynamon J, Labropoulos N, Haughton SH. Catheter-directed thrombolysis for lower extremity deep venous thrombosis: report of a national multicenter registry. Radiology. 1999; 211(1): 39–49
[9] Enden T, Haig Y, Kløw NE, et al. CaVenT Study Group. Long-term outcome after additional catheter-directed thrombolysis versus standard treatment for acute iliofemoral deep vein thrombosis (the CaVenT study): a randomised controlled trial. Lancet. 2012; 379(9810):31–38

[10] Haig Y, Enden T, Slagsvold CE, Sandvik L, Sandset PM, Kløw NE. Determinants of early and long-term efficacy of catheter-directed thrombolysis in proximal deep vein thrombosis. J Vasc Interv Radiol. 2013; 24(1):17–24, quiz 26

[11] Mickley V, Schwagierek R, Rilinger N, Görich J, Sunder-Plassmann L. Left iliac venous thrombosis caused by venous spur: treatment with thrombectomy and stent implantation. J Vasc Surg. 1998; 28(3):492–497

[12] Vedantham S, Sista AK, Klein SJ, et al. Society of Interventional Radiology and Cardiovascular and Interventional Radiological Society of Europe Standards of Practice Committees. Quality improvement guidelines for the treatment of lower-extremity deep vein thrombosis with use of endovascular thrombus removal. J Vasc Interv Radiol. 2014; 25(9):1317–1325

[13] Sharifi M, Bay C, Skrocki L, Lawson D, Mazdeh S. Role of IVC filters in endovenous therapy for deep venous thrombosis: the FILTER-PEVI (filter implantation to lower thromboembolic risk in percutaneous endovenous intervention) trial. Cardiovasc Intervent Radiol. 2012; 35(6):1408–1413

[14] Kahn SR, Shbaklo H, Shapiro S, et al. SOX Trial Investigators. Effectiveness of compression stockings to prevent the post-thrombotic syndrome (the SOX Trial and Bio-SOX biomarker substudy): a randomized controlled trial. BMC Cardiovasc Disord. 2007; 7:21

10.3 Filter-Related Adverse Events and Thresholds

Boris Nikolic

Monitoring and evaluating inferior vena cava (IVC) filter-related adverse events should never be considered or analyzed in isolation, but be embedded into an adequately comprehensive quality improvement program. Additional parameters, such as appropriateness of indication and patient selection, adequacy of preprocedural preparation, postprocedural patient monitoring, and retrieval rate for temporary IVC filters are additional parameters that fundamentally affect quality. These factors may also be causally related to adverse event occurrences. Some examples are permanent IVC filter placement in a preprocedurally bacteremic patient (where a subsequently placed IVC filter acts as a constant nidus for ongoing infection), wrong patient IVC filter insertion, allergic reaction to contrast media administration due to failure of preprocedural review of such available history, filter malpositioning or filter embolization in patients with anatomic variations or mega vena cava, respectively, that could have been recognizable during additional preprocedural review of existing cross-sectional imaging, etc. Along similar lines, premature discharge of a patient that is not fully awake and alert after receiving moderate sedation or puncture site hematoma formation may result from inadequate postprocedural patient monitoring.

Potential access site–related adverse events in association with IVC filter insertion include bleeding (6–15%)[1] and thrombosis (3–10%),[2] although the true incidence in general—and for individual operators/facilities in particular—is largely uncertain given the variability of patient follow-up and probable lack of clinical manifestation in most patients. Arteriovenous fistula formation and incomplete filter opening during deployment are theoretical risks but without respective recent reporting of incidences of occurrence. Aside from filter misplacement within the IVC, nontarget filter deployment into the gonadal vein, superior mesenteric vein, aorta, and within the spinal canal have all been reported.[3,4,5,6,7] Other than a minor malposition near the target area, filter malpositioning seems an avoidable phenomenon with proper utilization of image guidance (intravenous cavography and intravascular ultrasound). Similarly, upside-down filter placement should be considered a never event in interventional radiology. Specific thresholds for potential IVC filter-related adverse events have previously been established by the Standards of Practice Committee of the Society of Interventional Radiology (▶ Table 10.1). Performance of an internal institutional investigation is usually recommended when any of these thresholds are exceeded. However, factors such as patient sampling/selection bias or device failure and specifics may well contribute to such a scenario and early assignment of blame to the operator is therefore generally misguided. An additional caveat for threshold application arises if a specific procedure is rare at an institution, so that individual adverse events have disproportionate impact on the overall procedural volume percentage, which may even be the case for IVC filter placement and/or removal at some facilities. Impact of specific device or patient-related factors may further compound analysis of additional potential adverse events such as filter tilt, caval wall perforation, filter fracture, pulmonary embolism recurrence, and IVC thrombus formation or occlusion, which would likewise complicate determination of corresponding specific thresholds, rendering such attempt arguably inappropriate at this time. At the same time, rigorous patient follow-up, reporting, and scientific study for all of these events is highly warranted, so that thresholds can be appropriately refined where they exist and operator-related influences can be scientifically uncovered where thresholds are currently lacking.

Over the last few years, much discussion has evolved around adverse events that may more

Table 10.1 Reported inferior vena cava filter complication rates

Complication	Reported rates (%)	Threshold (%)
Death	0.12	< 1
Filter embolization	0.1	1
Filter malposition	1–9	0
Access site occlusive thrombosis	3–10	3

Source: *Molvar C. Interior vena cava filtration in the management of venous thormboembolism: filtering the data. Semin Intervent Radiol. 2012; 29(3):204–217.*

commonly afflict some types of retrievable IVC filter, such as filter fractures, migration as well as embolization of filter parts or the entire devices, device tilt, and caval wall perforation.[8,9,10,11] For IVC filters that are implanted if only temporary protection from pulmonary embolism is needed, relevance and requirement of patient monitoring often extends many weeks beyond the immediate postprocedural recovery time. Lack of patient tracking and filter retrieval seems to be associated with generally higher frequencies of fracturing of filter material or caval wall perforation, at least for individual device types.[12,13] A number of adverse events including but not limited to fragment embolization to the right heart, pulmonary arterial system, pericardium, iliac vein, and kidney have all been reported. The sequelae of caval wall perforation and filter migration may cause symptoms such as back pain, retroperitoneal hematoma, lumbar artery pseudoaneurysm formation, or gastrointestinal injury.[13,14,15,16,17] Careful patient follow-up and introduction of dedicated filter retrieval clinics have therefore been advocated, implementation of which has been accompanied by the expected increases in reported filter retrieval rates.[18,19,20,21,22,23] Analysis of the MAUDE database seems to suggest that adverse events are significantly more frequent in retrievable IVC filters than in permanent IVC filters; however, more rigorous follow-up and higher reporting rates for retrievable filters may well account for or contribute to this finding.[24] Generalized judgment regarding retrievable IVC filters may frequently be inappropriate, given the differences in individual filter design, variability of reporting and reported rates of adverse events for individual filters, evolution of individual filters in terms of manufacturing process, required retrieval technique and needed supplies, as well as overwhelmingly lower levels of evidence in the currently existing body of literature, typically presented as retrospective, single-center studies.[25,26]

Benefits of retrieval of IVC filters that are designed and labeled for such procedure as soon as their presence is no longer indicated have been well documented, because longer filter dwell times have been associated with increased risks of DVT as well as device fractures, limb perforation, and migration for at least some filter types.[9,14,27,28,29,30] At the same time, successful filter removal has been accomplished after 6 months for a variety of filter types, because of which such longer dwell time alone should generally

not discourage retrieval attempts.[31,32,33] Specific parameters known to potentially complicate filter retrieval are filter tilt, IVC wall perforation, and fractured or intraretrieval fracturing of filter material, and advanced retrieval techniques may be required for device removal under these circumstances.[34] A larger portion of published literature is dedicated to description of such advanced retrieval techniques, which include bronchial forceps use, balloon disruption, loop snare technique, and laser assistance.[8,35,36] Lower incidences of strut penetration and filter tilt have been reported for Denali filters compared to Celect filters.[26] As advanced technique applications may be associated with a higher adverse event rate, a more cautious approach in utilization of these techniques seems prudent.[8] Adverse events described with filter retrieval include IVC intussusception and dissection, filter fracturing, and hemorrhage (MAUDE). The general rule is to exercise the best case-based judgement in deciding whether filter retrieval or leaving a given filter in situ has the lower risk-to-benefit ratio prevails here as much as elsewhere in the practice of medicine. Referring the patient to a high-volume center with vast experience in filter retrieval may sometimes be most advisable for these generally elective procedures.

Placement of filters in the suprarenal IVC and superior vena cava (SVC) has been described anecdotally and in smaller case series.[37] Meaningful generalized conclusions cannot be drawn from the currently existing literature, and the potential for adverse events may be partly similar to what has been described for IVC filters placed in the infrarenal position. IVC filter placement is rarely indicated in pediatric patients and is often performed in patients with very limited prognosis where filter removal may therefore not be required.

In summary, the myriad of existing filter types and rapid generational evolution of devices frequently limits generalized conclusions and comparability among filters. Placement of retrievable filters should be followed by rigorous follow-up and device removal—if possible—as soon as its use is no longer indicated. Filter retrieval should always be attempted in completeness and include efforts to retrieve fractured fragments, if feasible. Scientifically rigorous efforts to prove IVC filtration effectiveness on the basis of strong evidence seem to be one of the most challenging yet meaningful tasks at this time.

References

[1] Joels CS, Sing RF, Heniford BT. Complications of inferior vena cava filters. Am Surg. 2003; 69(8):654–659

[2] Caplin DM, Nikolic B, Kalva SP, Ganguli S, Saad WE, Zuckerman DA, Society of Interventional Radiology Standards of Practice Committee. Quality improvement guidelines for the performance of inferior vena cava filter placement for the prevention of pulmonary embolism. J Vasc Interv Radiol. 2011; 22(11):1499–1506

[3] Martin MJ, Blair KS, Curry TK, Singh N. Vena cava filters: current concepts and controversies for the surgeon. Curr Probl Surg. 2010; 47(7):524–618

[4] Cronin B, Nguyen L, Manecke G, Pretorius V, Banks D, Maus T. Foreign body located intraoperatively using transesophageal echocardiography. J Cardiothorac Vasc Anesth. 2014; 28(3):852–853

[5] Tan WP, Sherer BA, Khare N. Unfriendly filter: an unusual cause of hydronephrosis and hematuria. Urology. 2016; 87:e9–e10

[6] Cuadra SA, Sales CM, Lipson AC, Armstrong CA. Misplacement of a vena cava filter into the spinal canal. J Vasc Surg. 2009; 50(5):1170–1172

[7] Grewal S, Chamarthy MR, Kalva SP. Complications of inferior vena cava filters. Cardiovasc Diagn Ther. 2016; 6(6):632–641

[8] Al-Hakim R, Kee ST, Olinger K, Lee EW, Moriarty JM, McWilliams JP. Inferior vena cava filter retrieval: effectiveness and complications of routine and advanced techniques. J Vasc Interv Radiol. 2014; 25(6):933–939, quiz 940

[9] Kuo WT, Robertson SW, Odegaard JI, Hofmann LV. Complex retrieval of fractured, embedded, and penetrating inferior vena cava filters: a prospective study with histologic and electron microscopic analysis. J Vasc Interv Radiol. 2013; 24(5):622–630.e1, quiz 631

[10] Dinglasan LA, Trerotola SO, Shlansky-Goldberg RD, Mondschein J, Stavropoulos SW. Removal of fractured inferior vena cava filters: feasibility and outcomes. J Vasc Interv Radiol. 2012; 23(2):181–187

[11] Vijay K, Hughes JA, Burdette AS, et al. Fractured Bard Recovery, G2, and G2 express inferior vena cava filters: incidence, clinical consequences, and outcomes of removal attempts. J Vasc Interv Radiol. 2012; 23(2):188–194

[12] Durack JC, Westphalen AC, Kekulawela S, et al. Perforation of the IVC: rule rather than exception after longer indwelling times for the Günther Tulip and Celect retrievable filters. Cardiovasc Intervent Radiol. 2012; 35(2):299–308

[13] An T, Moon E, Bullen J, et al. Prevalence and clinical consequences of fracture and fragment migration of the Bard G2 filter: imaging and clinical follow-up in 684 implantations. J Vasc Interv Radiol. 2014; 25(6):941–948

[14] Hull JE, Han J, Giessel GM. Retrieval of the recovery filter after arm perforation, fracture, and migration to the right ventricle. J Vasc Interv Radiol. 2008; 19(7):1107–1111

[15] Kendirli MT, Sildiroglu O, Cage DL, Turba UC. Inferior vena cava filter presenting as chronic low back pain. Clin Imaging. 2012; 36(3):236–238

[16] Jehangir A, Rettew A, Shaikh B, et al. IVC filter perforation through the duodenum found after years of abdominal pain. Am J Case Rep. 2015; 16:292–295

[17] Skeik N, McEachen JC, Stockland AH, et al. Lumbar artery pseudoaneurysm caused by a Gunther Tulip inferior vena cava filter. Vasc Endovascular Surg. 2011; 45(8):756–760

[18] Minocha J, Idakoji I, Riaz A, et al. Improving inferior vena cava filter retrieval rates: impact of a dedicated inferior vena cava filter clinic. J Vasc Interv Radiol. 2010; 21(12):1847–1851

[19] Ko SH, Reynolds BR, Nicholas DH, et al. Institutional protocol improves retrievable inferior vena cava filter recovery rate. Surgery. 2009; 146(4):809–814, discussion 814–816

[20] Lynch FC. A method for following patients with retrievable inferior vena cava filters: results and lessons learned from the first 1,100 patients. J Vasc Interv Radiol. 2011; 22(11):1507–1512

[21] Rogers FB, Shackford SR, Miller JA, Wu D, Rogers A, Gambler A. Improved recovery of prophylactic inferior vena cava filters in trauma patients: the results of a dedicated filter registry and critical pathway for filter removal. J Trauma Acute Care Surg. 2012; 72(2):381–384

[22] Ryu RK, Parikh P, Gupta R, et al. Optimizing IVC filter utilization: a prospective study of the impact of interventional radiologist consultation. J Am Coll Radiol. 2012; 9(9):657–660

[23] Lee MJ, Valenti D, de Gregorio MA, Minocha J, Rimon U, Pellerin O. The CIRSE retrievable IVC filter registry: retrieval success rates in practice. Cardiovasc Intervent Radiol. 2015; 38(6):1502–1507

[24] Andreoli JM, Lewandowski RJ, Vogelzang RL, Ryu RK. Comparison of complication rates associated with permanent and retrievable inferior vena cava filters: a review of the MAUDE database. J Vasc Interv Radiol. 2014; 25(8):1181–1185

[25] Hoffer EK, Mueller RJ, Luciano MR, Lee NN, Michaels AT, Gemery JM. Safety and efficacy of the Gunther Tulip retrievable vena cava filter: midterm outcomes. Cardiovasc Intervent Radiol. 2013; 36(4):998–1005

[26] Bos AS, Tullius T, Patel M, et al. Indwelling and retrieval complications of Denali and Celect infrarenal vena cava filters. J Vasc Interv Radiol. 2016; 27(7):1021–1026

[27] Group PS, PREPIC Study Group. Eight-year follow-up of patients with permanent vena cava filters in the prevention of pulmonary embolism: the PREPIC (Prevention du Risque d'Embolie Pulmonaire par Interruption Cave) randomized study. Circulation. 2005; 112(3):416–422

[28] Mismetti P. Randomized trial assessing the efficacy of the partial interruption of the inferior vena cava by an optional vena caval filter in the prevention of the recurrence of pulmonary embolism. PREPIC 2 trial: prevention of embolic recurrences by caval interruption (prospective, multicentric, randomised, open trial). Rev Pneumol Clin. 2008; 64(6):328–331

[29] Tam MD, Spain J, Lieber M, Geisinger M, Sands MJ, Wang W. Fracture and distant migration of the Bard Recovery filter: a retrospective review of 363 implantations for potentially life-threatening complications. J Vasc Interv Radiol. 2012; 23(2):199–205.e1

[30] Zhou D, Moon E, Bullen J, Sands M, Levitin A, Wang W. Penetration of Celect inferior vena cava filters: retrospective review of CT scans in 265 patients. AJR Am J Roentgenol. 2014; 202(3):643–647

[31] Binkert CA, Sasadeusz K, Stavropoulos SW. Retrievability of the recovery vena cava filter after dwell times longer than 180 days. J Vasc Interv Radiol. 2006; 17(2, Pt 1):299–302

[32] Lynch FC, Kekulawela S. Removal of the G2 filter: differences between implantation times greater and less than 180 days. J Vasc Interv Radiol. 2009; 20(9):1200–1209

[33] Zhu X, Tam MD, Bartholomew J, Newman JS, Sands MJ, Wang W. Retrievability and device-related complications of the G2 filter: a retrospective study of 139 filter retrievals. J Vasc Interv Radiol. 2011; 22(6):806–812

[34] Dinglasan LA, Oh JC, Schmitt JE, Trerotola SO, Shlansky-Goldberg RD, Stavropoulos SW. Complicated inferior vena cava filter retrievals: associated factors identified at preretrieval CT. Radiology. 2013; 266(1):347–354

[35] Stavropoulos SW, Dixon RG, Burke CT, et al. Embedded inferior vena cava filter removal: use of endobronchial forceps. J Vasc Interv Radiol. 2008; 19(9):1297–1301

[36] Stavropoulos SW, Ge BH, Mondschein JI, Shlansky-Goldberg RD, Sudheendra D, Trerotola SO. Retrieval of tip-embedded inferior vena cava filters by using the endobronchial forceps technique: experience at a single institution. Radiology. 2015; 275(3):900–907

[37] Owens CA, Bui JT, Knuttinen MG, Gaba RC, Carrillo TC. Pulmonary embolism from upper extremity deep vein thrombosis and the role of superior vena cava filters: a review of the literature. J Vasc Interv Radiol. 2010; 21(6):779–787

Index

Note: Page numbers set **bold** or *italic* indicate headings or figures, respectively.